How To Create A Medical Surveillance Program

How To Create A Medical Surveillance Program

An Example of a Program

Thomas M. Socha

Writers Club Press
San Jose New York Lincoln Shanghai

How To Create A Medical Surveillance Program
An Example of a Program

Writers Club Press
an imprint of iUniverse.com, Inc.

For information address:
iUniverse.com, Inc.
5220 S 16th, Ste. 200
Lincoln, NE 68512
www.iuniverse.com

ISBN: 0-595-20082-6

Printed in the United States of America

In memory of all those who lost their lives on September 11, 2001 at the hands of terrorists.

God Bless America

Contents

SCOPE

REQUIREMENTS OF A MEDICAL SURVEILLANCE PROGRAM

Workplace Exposures

OCCUPATIONAL EVALUATION TYPES

Preplacement or Baseline

Periodic

Termination

OCCUPATIONAL MEDICAL EXAMINATION

Background Information

Occupational Medical Surveillance

Use of Disease Questionnaires

OCCUPATIONAL MEDICAL EXAMINATION PROCESS

Identifying Workers Who Need Occupational Medical
Examinations

DETERMINING EVALUATION CONTENT AND DEVELOPING
PROTOCOLS

PERFORMING THE EVALUATION

RECORD KEEPING (DOCUMENTING EXAMINATION
RESULTS)

INFORMING THE WORKER OF EXAMINATION RESULTS

LIST OF TABLES

PREFACE

This book uses the May 1998, *Department of Defense Occupational Health Surveillance Manual* as an outline. Much of Chapter 1 and Notes are taken from this manual. Common medical surveillance programs which are not discussed in this book are the Lead and Asbestos programs and the Occupational Safety and Health Administration Table-Z listings.

ACKNOWLEDGEMENTS

I like to acknowledge the following institutions:

Arizona State University;
The U.S. Department of Defense;
Oakland University;
University of California at Davis;
University of Michigan, and
University of Missouri–Columbia

INTRODUCTION

The purpose of this book is to provide a guideline for the Medical Surveillance Program (MSP). It is also intended to help occupational health professionals and others recognize and evaluate health risks associated with specific workplace exposures.

The Office of Environmental Health and Safety (EHS) should administer the MSP. The program prevents occupational illness and injury among employees by "monitoring" certain health indicators that give clues to potential exposures and injury risks. Workplace risks for exposure or injury can generally be anticipated, recognized, evaluated, and controlled through conventional safety and industrial hygiene methods. These are not perfect; however, medical surveillance detects inapparent or unsuspected cases before they can become serious or lead to permanent injury.

Employee medical surveillance is a strategy for optimizing the health status of persons who work in settings where hazards exist. Medical surveillance involves a careful search for unexpected outcomes that might herald new or uncontrolled hazards in the workplace. It most often refers to the systematic collection, analysis and dissemination of health information on groups of workers. For medical surveillance to be an effective warning mechanism, it must be connected to preventive safety and health actions.

Medical surveillance is often called "medical monitoring", because certain health parameters are monitored that correspond to specific occupational risks. For instance, if an employee has occupational exposure to lead, either through paint-removal operations, or handling of lead bricks for radiation shielding, or application of lead-containing pottery glazes, their respirator or other protective measures, may fail or they may receive an overexposure. This overexposure may be inapparent, even though it is hazardous to their long-term health. They should receive medical monitoring for that exposure risk through yearly blood draw and blood-lead-level analysis. Also, a negative-pressure respirator will place a cardiovascular stress in the employee that presents a health risk if they have a medical impairment. A physical examination, abbreviated just for this risk, will verify that the employee is physically fit to perform their work while wearing a respirator. This testing includes pulmonary function testing to verify the employee's lungs are healthy and can provide enough oxygen under work and respirator stresses. An approved occupational medical service provider provides the testing. These are just two examples of a number of medical protocols designed to address the specific work conditions and potential risks of various occupations.

Occupational health problems can be prevented or their effects minimized if identified early. However, occupational medical examinations are preventive only if the workers at risk are properly identified and appropriately evaluated, and the results are used to modify exposure through work practices, process changes, engineering controls, administrative controls, personal protective equipment, or worker placement.

The approved occupational medical provider employs physicians and nurses licensed and certified in occupational medicine and its various specialty functions. The provider works with ESH to assure that all testing is administered properly, medical physician's determinations are delivered in a timely fashion, and records are adequately maintained. These activities are regulated by standards set by the federal Department of Labor's Occupational Safety and Health Administration (OSHA).

Chapter 1: Requirements of a Medical Surveillance Program

The Medical Surveillance Program (better know as OSHA Physical Exam) Through the program employees are monitored for certain health indicators, depending on their job assignments. These "indicators" medical tests informs EHS if the employee is fit to perform their duties and will also give us early detection of illness or injury that may have been a result of work, before the incurred condition becomes serious.

SCOPE

This book is intended to assist in the administration of the medical surveillance program. Employees covered by this program are those assigned to jobs where there may be potential exposure to hazardous material/conditions, or employees using equipment that requires medical clearance. Temporary as well as permanent employees may be included in the program.

Administration of the Medical Surveillance Program can be functionally divided into four areas:

1. Identification of at-risk employees via job title or tasks;

2. Setting standards of testing reporting;

3. Medical administration–tracking, scheduling of appointments, and internal recordkeeping and

4. Continuous screening, auditing, and quality assurance for the various programs aspects.

If you are determined to be covered under the regulatory requirements for medical surveillance, you will be notified through your supervisor and entered into the program.

The confidentiality of your medical records and tests results is protected under the law. The company or EHS only receives a simple physician's determination as to whether or not an employee is physically fit to work under the stress presented by their work environment and personal protective equipment. The EHS receives no test results or diagnoses concerning the employee's general health or particular conditions. If an employee is determined not to be physically fit for a particular type of work or task, this will be discussed in detail with employee and noted as a restriction on the physician's determination.

REQUIREMENTS OF A MEDICAL SURVEILLANCE PROGRAM

Workplace Exposures

Industrial hygiene surveys of workplace must identify all potential exposures and other worker safety and health risks, and establish complete workplace exposure profiles.

Should potentially hazardous agents not covered in this Manual be identified, promptly notify EHS to initiate appropriate hazard evaluation (refer to Appendix A).

OCCUPATIONAL EVALUATION TYPES

Preplacement or Baseline

These examinations are performed before placement in a specific job to assess, if the worker will be able to perform the job capably and safely, to determine if the worker meets any established physical standards, and to obtain baseline measurements for future comparison

Periodic

These examinations are conducted at scheduled intervals. Periodic examinations may include an interval history, physical examination, and/or clinical and biological screening tests. The scope of these examinations is determined after consideration of the information contained in this Manual, professional practice standards, regulatory guidance, and any other relevant factors.

Termination

There are two kinds of termination examinations.

Termination-of-Employment. These examinations are designed to assess pertinent aspects of the worker's health when the employee leaves employment. Documentation of examination results may be beneficial in assessing the relationship of any future medical problems to an exposure in the workplace. This is particularly applicable to those conditions that are chronic or that may have long latency periods. Some Federal regulations require termination of employment examinations (e.g. asbestos, 29 CFR 1910.1001). [1]

Termination of Exposure These examinations are performed when exposure to a specific hazard has ceased. Exposure to specific hazards may cease when a worker is reassigned, a process is changed, or the worker leaves employment. Terminations of exposure examinations are most beneficial when the health effect being screened for is likely to be present at the time exposure ceases.

Some Federal regulations require termination of exposure examinations (29 CFR 1910.120). [2]

OCCUPATIONAL MEDICAL EXAMINATION

Background Information

The primary reasons for conducting occupational medical examinations are listed in the following sections. When performing an examination (or constructing an examination protocol), the practitioner must understand the reasons for obtaining each historical item, performing each physical examination procedure, and ordering each laboratory test. This understanding is essential for the practitioner to know how to properly perform the examination, investigate abnormalities, and formulate appropriate medical recommendations.

Occupational Medical Surveillance

Occupational medical surveillance examinations provide baseline and periodic measurements to detect abnormalities in workers who are exposed to work-related health hazards early enough to prevent or limit disease progression by exposure modification or medical intervention. Medical surveillance examinations are secondary prevention measures. They are effective only if useful screening techniques (history questionnaires, medical exams, or lab tests) are available to identify abnormalities in the target organ system at a stage when modifying exposure or providing medical treatment can arrest progression or prevent recurrence.

Much of the information in this Manual is presented to assist health professionals in identifying known work-related health hazards, the target organ system, specific health effects, and useful screening tests.

Use of Disease Questionnaires

Comparison of the results from previous years with present results provides the best method for detecting a general deterioration in health when toxic signs and symptoms are measured subjectively. In this way recall bias does not affect the results of the analysis. Consequently,

OSHA has determined that the findings of the medical and work histories should be kept in a standardized form for comparison of the year-to-year results (refer to Appendix B).

OCCUPATIONAL MEDICAL EXAMINATION PROCESS

Identifying Workers Who Need Occupational Medical Examinations

There are three ways to identify workers at risk of work-related health problems: by job title, by workplace, and by individual exposure.

Job Title. Job title and description characterize the basic tasks, hazardous exposures, and health outcomes likely to be experienced by the majority of workers in a specific occupational group. This type of grouping assumes all workers will have similar job demands, experience similar stresses, have the same exposures to hazardous agents, and suffer the same health effects.

Workplace. Workplace characterizes the hazardous agents present in the workplace and assumes all workers assigned to that workplace are potentially exposed to the levels of hazards found at the time the workplace was evaluated.

Individual Exposure. Individual exposure quantifies job demands, stresses, and hazardous exposures for each individual.

Each method has limitations. Likewise, any standardized examination protocol developed using a single method to identify the workers at risk will be limited. To minimize these limitations, a combination of these methods is recommended.

DETERMINING EVALUATION CONTENT AND DEVELOPING PROTOCOLS

Installation occupational health and safety personnel are jointly responsible for identifying work areas where workers need medical examinations because of specific hazardous exposures. Local occupational medical personnel establish examination content and frequency based on an understanding of the job demands, exposures to the workers, the medical effects of specific exposures, and the impact of specific medical conditions on job performance and safety, and legal and regulatory requirements.

Examination protocols may include employee health promotion and personnel programs. Local medical personnel must be aware of collective bargaining agreements and support agreements that entitle specific employee groups to health benefit programs or other medical benefits. If medical examinations are deemed inappropriate or of little value, documentation of the rationale used in making this decision shall be maintained locally.

The following list summarizes factors to consider when determining examination content and developing examination protocols.

1. Specific job tasks and/or requirements.

2. Workplace risk factors (exposures).

3. Physical agents.

4. Chemical agents.

5. Biological agents.

6. Other.

7. Personal risk factors (medical status).

8. Target organ systems and potential health risks.

9. Potential public health and safety impact.

10. Legal and regulatory requirements.

11. Employee health promotion and personnel programs.

PERFORMING THE EVALUATION

The occupational medicine practitioner takes a targeted medical history based on complaints and risk factors, does a review of systems, and then performs selected physical examinations and laboratory tests to characterize the status of specific organ systems. In some cases, a standard examination protocol (historical questionnaire and lab tests) may be administered to a group of workers with similar specific health risks.

Workers receiving occupational medical examinations can have health conditions that can affect their job performance or indicate a problem in the workplace. Determining a particular worker's fitness and risk for a particular job and identifying work-related medical conditions requires medical judgment by a practitioner knowledgeable of the worker's working conditions and job demands.

RECORD KEEPING (DOCUMENTING EXAMINATION RESULTS)

Occupational medical surveillance examinations shall be recorded and maintained. All results should be recorded in employee's medical records. Standard or customized forms may be used or developed to aid in collecting and recording occupational medical information.

INFORMING THE WORKER OF EXAMINATION RESULTS

All workers must be informed of the results of their occupational medical examination (even if all results are normal) as soon as possible following completion. Documentation of patient notification should be noted in the medical record. All personnel with significant abnormalities must be further evaluated or referred for evaluation as appropriate. One of the primary reasons for performing occupational medical examinations is to detect job-related abnormalities at an early stage to reverse or halt progression by modifying exposure. If abnormalities are not fully evaluated and reviewed, potential opportunities for prevention are lost (refer to Appendix C).

COUNSELING AND EDUCATION CONCERNING IDENTIFIED HEALTH RISKS

Medical personnel shall inform workers receiving occupational medical examinations of any specific health risks present in the work environment. The extent of the information provided to the worker will vary depending on the nature of the hazards and health status of the worker. This should not be interpreted as a requirement to establish formal education programs in the medical facility to inform every worker of their specific potential health risks. This may be appropriate in some cases. However, in most cases a short verbal explanation of the reasons for the examination and the types of health effects being screened for is sufficient.

MEDICAL DETERMINATIONS AND RECOMMENDATIONS

A medical examination alone cannot determine an individual's ability to perform the essential duties of a particular position. The responsibility for making this determination rests solely with the appointing official. Employment-related decisions involving health are fundamentally managerial, not medical.

Medical information may be an essential element in determining an individual's suitability for job tasks. However, management has the obligation to consider issues that are not strictly medical (e.g., reasonable accommodation or assessment of undue hardship on the operation of the agency's operations).

The role of occupational medical personnel in addressing employment decisions is limited to determining whether the individual meets the medical requirements of the position and can, from a medical standpoint, perform the job capably and safely.

To assist managers in making employment and placement decisions, medical determinations should fall in one of the following three categories.

Qualified–The individual meets the medical requirements of the position and is (from a medical standpoint) capable of performing the required tasks. Allowing the individual to perform the job will not pose a significant risk to personal health and safety or the health and safety of others.

Qualified with Restriction–The individual meets the medical requirements of the position and is capable of performing the job without risk to personal health or others only with some accommodation or restriction. (When this determination is made, the practitioner should provide a list of recommended accommodations or restrictions and the expected duration of this requirement and therapeutic or risk-avoiding benefit.)

Not Qualified–The individual is incapable of performing essential tasks, will be unsafe, or fails to meet medical requirements for the job (refer to Appendix C).

Recommended Disqualification Procedure

A disqualifying or not qualified medical determination is legitimate if:

1. A medical condition prevents the worker from performing the essential functions of the job and no reasonable accommodation would enable the worker to perform the job.

2. Allowing the worker to perform the job would endanger the health or safety of other workers or the public.

3. Placing (or retaining) the individual in the job poses a significant risk to the worker's personal health or safety.

4. The individual fails to meet a medical standard or physical requirement for placement in the position.

Determination of Unsuitability to Work

The examining practitioner should prepare a case summary on all workers determined to be medically unsuited for their job and file this case summary in the workers medical record. The appointing official must be informed of the disqualifying recommendation. The case summary, as confidential medical information, should be provided to management only when necessary and authorized. The following information should be included in all case summaries:

Diagnosis. The diagnosis must be justified in accordance with established diagnostic criteria.

History. The history of the disqualifying condition(s) including references to findings from previous examinations, treatment, and responses to treatment.

Clinical findings. The clinical findings including results of any laboratory tests, x-rays, or special evaluations performed.

Prognosis. The prognosis must clearly state the medical basis for concluding that the individual is incapable or unsafe, plans or recommendations for future treatment, and an estimate of the expected date of full or partial recovery. If recovery is not expected this should also be clearly indicated. The prognosis must also include an explanation of the impact of the medical condition on overall activities both on and off the job, the reason(s) why restrictions or accommodations will not enable the individual to perform the job, and an explanation of the medical basis for any conclusions.

Chapter 2: Health Care Workers

Health care facilities may present a number of hazards for health care workers (HCWs). Paragraphs a through d provides a partial listing of possible hazards in the hospital worksite.

HAZARDOUS DESCRIPTION

Hazardous Drugs

Hazardous drugs are those drugs, whether considered cytotoxic or not, that have proven genotoxicity, carcinogenicity, teratogenicity or fertility impairment, or produce serious organ or other toxic manifestations at low doses in experimental animals or treated patients. Essentially all chemotherapeutic agents and a significant number of the anti-viral agents are included in this category. Worker exposure to these agents occurs during drug preparation, administration, and disposal under the OSHA Technical Manual Directive[3].

Mycobacterium tuberculosis

Mycobacterium tuberculosis (TB) is an aerosol-spread organism that is a known cause of human infection. Transmission of M. tuberculosis from individuals with respiratory infection is a known risk to patients and HCWs in health-care facilities. Historically respiratory tuberculosis infections were treatable with anti-tuberculous medication. Recently the organism has developed resistance to standard anti-tuberculous medication and this resistant organism is referred to as MDR-TB (multi-drug resistant tuberculosis). This emergence of drug-resistant organisms, along the with the difficulty in identifying and diagnosing the tuberculosis infection, especially in individuals with other underlying diseases such as AIDS, has increased the risk of exposure to TB for HCWs under the guidelines[4]. TB infection in humans can be categorized as "latent" or active. Latent TB infection is an asymptomatic condition characterized by a positive purified protein tuberculin (PPD) skin test. Individuals with latent TB may or may not have chest x-ray findings consistent with "old TB." On the other hand, cough, sputum production, fever, night sweats, and weight loss usually characterize active respiratory pulmonary TB infection. Typically, if the infected individual has an otherwise intact immune system, the TB skin test is positive and the chest x-ray will reveal evidence of the infection. Prevention of the spread of TB is through the early identification and isolation of infected individuals and the use of respiratory protection by the HCWs. If the HCW is provided respiratory protection they must also be enrolled in the Respiratory Protection Program (see Chapter 5).

Other Chemical and Physical Hazards

Health Care Workers frequently encounter numerous other workplace hazards. The biomechanical hazards of lifting patients and pushing food and laundry carts are a common cause of low back pain and injury in the health care setting. Heat and noise hazards can also be found in mechanical spaces, laundries and kitchens. Many chemicals are used in the hospital work environment. Individual OSHA standards govern the medical screening for workers exposed to ethylene oxide and formaldehyde, but other common hospital chemicals, such glutaraldehyde, are not covered by any specific regulation. A recent addition to the list of hospital workplace hazards is exposure to airborne latex particles from gloves and other products made from latex. These latex particles have been identified as a cause of allergic reactions in both patients and sensitized workers[5].

Blood-borne Pathogens

Requirements for the medical aspects of the Blood-borne pathogens program, including vaccination against hepatitis B virus, are found in Chapter 4.

EXPOSURE LIMITS

Not applicable.

TARGET ORGAN(S) AND POTENTIAL HEALTH EFFECTS

See Hazardous Descriptions in this chapter.

CRITERIA FOR ENTRY INTO MEDICAL SURVEILLANCE PROGRAM

Criteria for entry into the medical programs for the OSHA-mandated Blood-borne Pathogens and Respiratory Protection programs are provided in Chapters 4 and 5. The OSHA Technical Manual chapter on controlling occupational exposures to hazardous drugs, recommends that those employees potentially exposed to hazardous drugs be enrolled in medical surveillance programs under the OSHA Technical Manual Directive[3] .In 1994 the Centers for Disease Control and Prevention published "Guidelines for Preventing the Transmission of Mycobacterium tuberculosis in Health-Care Facilities, 1994" (MMWR volume 43 RR-13, Oct 28, 1994) [4]. These guidelines outlined the tuberculosis program recommended for health-care facilities and the requirements for TB skin testing in HCWs.

SURVEILLANCE FREQUENCY

Pre-placement evaluations are indicated for all HCWs with potential hazardous exposures. The frequency of follow-up evaluations is based upon type, duration and risk of exposure. Health care facilities at high-risk for tuberculosis exposure may need to conduct TB screening every three-six months or as needed following known exposures. Otherwise, periodic screening is generally done annually. Examinations following acute exposures and at the termination of employment are also recommended for HCWs exposed to hazardous drugs. Recommendations for post-exposure prophylaxix for HIV exposed workers are provided in reference[6].

MEDICAL AND OCCUPATIONAL HISTORY

The medical and occupational history should be tailored to the type of HCW exposure.

All HCWs should be asked about medical conditions that may suppress their immune system, including underlying chronic medical conditions, (i.e., chronic renal failure, diabetes mellitus), use of corticosteriods, and use of immune suppressive agents (refer to Appendix B).

Verification of immunizations or documentation of antibodies to specific viruses is required of all HCWs. In addition to hepatitis B, immunization or immunity to rubella, measles, mumps and varicella (chicken pox) may be required or recommended[7].

History of exposure to tuberculosis and history of results of prior TB skin testing.

History of allergic dermatitis and specifically history of allergy to latex products.

History of use or ability to wear respirator (TB and Respiratory Protection Program).

Reproductive status (specifically for female HCWs—if they are currently pregnant).

PHYSICAL EXAMINATION

The physical examination requirements, like the medical/occupational history requirements, will need to be based upon the toxic effects of the potential exposure and the need for respiratory protection or other personal protective equipment. For HCWs with potential exposure to hazardous drugs, a complete examination with emphasis on the skin, mucous membranes, cardiopulmonary system, lymphatic system, and liver is recommended.

LABORATORY

Immunizations, as indicated, or verification of immunity if required.

TB skin testing as recommended by CDC guidelines[8].

Other laboratory testing as indicated by history and physical examination.

Annual influenza vaccination for health care workers is recommended by the Centers for Disease Control and Prevention[9].

For HCWs with exposure to hazardous drugs, a complete blood count with differential white blood cell count, liver function tests, blood urea nitrogen, creatinine, and urinalysis are recommended. The frequency of this testing may be from every year to every three years and should be determined by exposure, worker history and discretion of occupational medicine physician under the OSHA Technical Manual Directive[3].

OTHER ELEMENTS

Refer to Chapter 4 for requirements for the exposure to blood-borne pathogens. Hepatitis B Vaccination Declination Form should be completed and filed in the HCWs medical record if the HCW declines to receive the hepatitis B vaccination series.

Table 2-1 Requirements For Health Care Workers

Requirements For Health Care Workers	
Pre-placement exam	Yes- If based upon the toxic effects of the potential exposure and the need for respiratory protection or other personal protective equipment. A questionnaire is necessary.
Periodic exam	Yes – See Pre- Placement exam.
Emergency/exposure Examination and Tests	Yes
Termination exam	Yes – Following acute exposures and at the termination of employment are also recommended for HCWs exposed to hazardous drugs.
Examination includes special emphasis on these body systems	Blood, skin, and respiratory system.
Work and medical history	Yes
Chest x-ray	As determine by a physician or other licensed health care professional.
Pulmonary function test (PFT)	Yes, if using a respiratory or determined by a physician or other licensed health care professional
Other required tests	Immunizations, as indicated, or verification of immunity if required. Vaccination against hepatitis B virus. TB skin testing as recommended by CDC guidelines.
Evaluation of ability to wear A respirator	Yes – if required.
Additional Tests if deemed necessary	The CDC recommends annual influenza vaccination for health care workers.
Written medical opinion	Yes
Employee counseling re: exam results, Conditions of increased risk	Yes
Medical removal plan	No

Chapter 3: Animal Care Handlers

HAZARD DESCRIPTION

Animal handlers who work with or around wild, domestic or laboratory animals may be at risk for a number of infectious diseases spread by or in association with animals. In addition to the infectious hazards, small proteins from animal dander or urine may be the cause of allergic reactions in sensitized individuals. Work with or around animals can also expose the worker to biomechanical hazards associated with lifting cages or feedbags and physical trauma secondary to bites and scratches from animals. Numerous infectious diseases (zoonoses) can be spread through contact with animals, animal excretions or biologic material. Rabies is a well-known animal-related infectious disease but other less well-known diseases, such as Q-fever, brucellosis, and herpes B virus can be spread from animals to humans. Allergies to animals or animal products can produce a spectrum of allergic responses from common allergic conjunctivitis and rhinitis to life threatening asthma.[10]

Zoonoses are infectious diseases transmitted from animals to man. Most animals used in research do not pose a risk to people handling them because whenever possible, disease-free animals are utilized as research subjects. Nevertheless, on rare occasions, animal handlers can contract diseases from research animals. A few examples of zoonoses reported in animal handlers are provided in Table 3-2. Primates, wild animals, dogs, cats and some farm animals can carry diseases that pose the greatest risks to humans. Therefore, the health program for people working with these species is somewhat different than the program for people working with rodents.

Injury from animal bites or scratches present the greatest risk to animal handlers because many pathogens are found on the oral mucosa or in the saliva of laboratory animals. For example, two serious zoonoses that are relatively rare but often fatal are rabies and Herpes B encephalitis. Rabies can be carried by a number of wild mammals such as bats, raccoons and skunks, but may also occur in domestic carnivores such as dogs. By comparison, the Herpes B virus is carried only by certain species of nonhuman primates, principally macaques such as rhesus and cynomolgus monkeys. Both diseases are transmitted through bites or scratches from infected animals. Less serious diseases can result following scratches from cats and bites from rodents.

Many species of laboratory animals have been implicated in allergy problems. Dander, serum, urine, and saliva are just some of the materials that can induce an allergic response in an animal handler who is sensitized to these animal products. Allergic responses generally are seen immediately after handling an animal but may not appear for several hours after exposure. Sneezing, tearing and red, swollen eyes are typical signs but other responses such as a rash, wheal, hives or other type of skin inflammation also may be seen.

EXPOSURE LIMITS

There are no exposure limits for this occupational category.

TARGET ORGAN(S) AND POTENTIAL HEALTH EFFECTS

The target organs and potential health effects will depend upon the hazards to which the employee is exposed. All infectious diseases can affect the immune and lymphatic system; sensitizing animal proteins can affect the respiratory system through the induction or aggravation of allergic rhinitis and asthma; and the known teratogenic agents such as Toxoplasma gondii can affect the reproductive system or reproduction.

CRITERIA FOR ENTRY INTO MEDICAL SURVEILLANCE PROGRAM

There are no mandatory criteria for entrance into medical surveillance programs for individuals exposed to animals. This program is designed for personnel who have occupational exposure to animals including: the direct care of animals or their living areas; or the direct contact with animals (live or sacrificed), their viable tissues, body fluids, or wastes.

If a determination is made that you are eligible for participation in the program, you will be assigned to one of three risk categories based upon the species of animals with which you are or will be working, and the potential risks to you.

Those categories are:

Risk Category 1:	Rodents (rats, mice, hamsters, guinea pigs, etc.), rabbits, birds, aquatics (reptiles, or amphibians).
Risk Category 2:	Domestic carnivores (cats, dogs), livestock (sheep, cattle, swine, goats), or any wild caught mammal except non-human primates
Risk Category 3:	Non-human primates.

Risk Category 1: Rodents (rats, mice, hamsters, guinea pigs, etc.), rabbits, birds, aquatics (reptiles, or amphibians). **Risk Category 2:** Domestic carnivores (cats, dogs), livestock (sheep, cattle, swine, goats), or any wild caught mammal except non-human primates. **Risk Category 3:** Non-human primates.

The content of the medical surveillance program, including content of screening or requirements for immunizations, is based upon the Risk Category.

NOTE:

Pregnant woman should have no work contact with cats.

SURVEILLANCE FREQUENCY

Pre-placement evaluations are recommended for all animal handlers. The periodic examination frequency is based upon Risk Category and the need for immunizations. If periodic evaluations are necessary (i.e. zoonoses questionnaire), they are generally done annually (refer to Appendix D).

MEDICAL AND OCCUPATIONAL HISTORY

The medical and occupational history should concentrate on those conditions or exposures that may place the worker at increased risk for infection (refer to Appendix D). The following specific areas should be emphasized.

History of medical conditions associated with suppression of the immune system, including underlying chronic medical conditions, (i.e., chronic renal failure, diabetes mellitus), use of corticosteroids, and use of immune suppressive agents.

The medical history questionnaire asks for verification of immunizations, including tetanus.

History of allergies, including atopy, dermatitis, allergic rhinitis, asthma, and sensitivity to latex products.

Reproductive status of worker (specifically current pregnancy for female animal handlers.)

PHYSICAL EXAMINATION

Pre-placement examination requirements and annual medical screening for animal handlers may vary by Risk Category and job description. All risk categories should have vital signs and a review of their medical history. Additional requirements include rabies and other immunizations, and Toxoplasmosis and Q-fever titers.

Laboratory animal care personnel, and others to whom this program is applicable, should receive general medical examinations at the time of employment to establish the status of health and to evaluate exceptional risk due to underlying conditions or disease. Thereafter, the EHS (see Table 3-1) should conduct medical examinations annually during the individual's employment.

The frequency of exams may be increased, and/or specific diagnostic procedures may be added to the general exam, in cases where specific known hazards exist.

The examination should include the following:

1. The animal resource supervisor in conjunction with Environmental Health and Safety will provide the examining physician with a description of the employee's duties, including:

- The animal species contacted.
- The toxic, biologic and radiologic agents under investigation.

2. Tuberculin Tests should be conducted as a part of the general physical exam at the time of employment and annually thereafter. Employees who are positive for the skin test may be required to have chest x-rays at the discretion of the attending physician.

3. Immunizations:

- All personnel working with animals should be immunized against tetanus.
- Those working with mammals that are raised in other than a laboratory setting should be immunized against rabies virus.
- The animal resource director, the program's principal investigator and the physician should consider use of available vaccines, bacterins or immune sera for specific biologic hazards.

4. Reference sera should be maintained and updated routinely for all personnel working with animals or fresh animal tissues.

5. The examining physician must provide a written opinion to the employer, including:

- Any medical condition of the employee that would increase risk of material impairment of health.
- Any medical condition of the employee that requires further examination or treatment.

6. The physician's original report shall be sent to the Office of Environmental Health and Safety, to satisfy record keeping requirements. This office will send copies to the appropriate animal resource supervisor.

NOTE: The employer must provide a copy of the physician's opinion to the employee.

ADDITIONAL STUDIES

All Risk Categories: Tetanus immunization history and immunization update as indicated.

Additional for Risk Category 2: toxoplasmosis titer for females of childbearing age with exposure to cats; rabies prophylaxis if exposure warrants; and Q-fever titer if exposure warrants.

Additional for Risk Category 3: rubeola titer/immunization if exposure warrants, and tuberculosis screening by skin test if indicated.

OTHER ELEMENTS

Rabies immunization. Individuals who should receive pre-exposure prophylaxis with human diploid cell rabies vaccine (HDCV) include: those working directly with rabies virus; those having direct contact with animals in quarantine; those having exposure to potentially infected animal body organs or performing post-mortem examinations on animals with a history of poorly defined neurological disorders; those having the responsibility for capturing or destroying wild animals; or those having large animal (Risk Category 2) contact where a potential for exposure exists. Serological monitoring is performed annually on all HDCV recipients with the exception of the first year when the primary series is given. Booster doses are administered to employees with inadequate titers unless they have a history of a hypersensitivity reaction to the vaccine.

Toxoplasmosis titer. Women of childbearing age who are occupationally exposed to cats and/or their waste should be screened for toxoplasmosis and receive appropriate health education regarding the risk of this disease during pregnancy. Every effort should be made to arrange temporary job reassignment while a susceptible employee is pregnant.

Q fever titer. Employees at risk of exposure to Q fever include those with direct contact with Coxiella burnetti and those who handle or use products of parturition (placenta, amniotic fluid, blood or soiled bedding) from infected sheep, be assessed for the likelihood of developing chronic sequelae of Q fever should they acquire the disease. Individuals susceptible include those who are immunosuppressed and/or have valvular or congenital heart problems.

Specific immunizations. Other specific immunizations and antibody titers should be given or obtained on all animal-handlers working with specific agents or with infected or potentially infected animals.

Storage or banking of serum samples is not required except when determined to be appropriate and beneficial for the potential exposures encountered. If serum samples are stored, it is imperative that proper labeling and storage are available[11].

Table 3-1: Animal Handlers Medical Surveillance Program: Physical Exams

Risk Category Code / Physical Exam	1	2	3
Type of Animal Contact	Small Animals (birds, rodents, rabbits, fish, amphibians, reptiles)	Large animals (cats, dogs, livestock, wild animals expect primates	Non-human Primates
Complete Medical Exam	Pre-placement	Pre-placement	Pre-placement
Tuberculin Skin Test (PPD)[1]	---	---	Pre-placement and every 6 months
Chest Roentgenogram	---	---	Pre-placement and as recommended by physician if PPD conversion
Rabies Vaccines	---	Pre-placement	Pre-placement
Rabies Booster	---	Every 2 years	Every 2 years
Diphtheria/Tetanus	Every 10 years	Every 10 years	Every 10 years
Annual Questionnaire	Yes and interview[2]	Yes and interview[2]	Yes and interview[2]
Other	---	Provide information on Q fever to livestock users / Toxoplasmosis titer for females of child-bearing age with exposure to cats; / Rabies prophylaxis if exposure warrants	Rubeola titer/immunization if exposure warrants

[1] Individuals with a previous history of positive TB reactions will be issued a semi-annual questionnaire regarding possible symptoms of Tuberculosis
[2] Interviews will be conducted on campus by qualified personnel from the Health Care Provider.

Table 3-2: Selected Zoonoses Reported in Animal Handlers

DISEASE	SPECIES	MODE OF TRANSMISSION	SYMPTOMS IN HUMANS	CONTROL
Toxoplasmosis	Cats	Oocysts present in feces	Influenza like signs potential birth defects	Pregnant woman should have no work contact with cats; protective clothing for others
Rabies	Dog, cats, wild animals	Bite wound or contact with infected saliva	Headache, rise in temperature pain from the bite wound, death	Vaccine
Herpes B	Primates	Bite wounds, virus shed in saliva and urogential secretions	Fever, nausea, death	Protective clothing proper handling and; restraint techniques
Q-Fever	Sheep, goats, cattle	Organism present in placental secretions and fluids	Fever, chills, sweating, loss of appetite	Protective clothing; special biocontainment practices
Rat Bite Fever	Rodents	Bite wounds	Wound inflammation, recurring fever, muscle pain, loss of appetite	Proper handling and restraint techniques; protective clothing
Lymphocytic choriomeningitis	Hamsters, mice	Organism present in feces, urine, nasal secretions, blood	Stiff neck, fever, muscle strain	Hand washing after animal contact, immediate cleansing and disinfection of wounds
Contagious Ecthyma	Sheep	Virus is in lesions in oral cavity and is transmitted in the saliva	Rash, blisters	Wear gloves
Tuberculosis	Primates	Organism present in respiratory secretions and is transmitted by aerosol	Often asymptomatic; cough fatigue, fever, weight loss, blood on sputum	Protective clothing; proper handling and restraint techniques

Chapter 4: Bloodborne Pathogens

HAZARDOUS DESCRIPTION

Certain pathogenic microorganisms can be found in the blood of infected individuals. For the purposes of this standard, OSHA is referring to these microorganisms as "bloodborne pathogens" and to the diseases that they cause as "bloodborne diseases." These bloodborne pathogens may be transmitted from the infected individual to other individuals by blood or certain other body fluids, for example, when intravenous drug users share blood-contaminated needles. Because it is the exposure to blood or other body fluids that carries the risk of infection, individuals whose occupational duties place them at risk of exposure to blood or other potentially infectious materials are also at risk of becoming infected with these bloodborne pathogens, developing disease and, in some cases, dying. Infected individuals are also capable of transmitting the pathogens to others.

The two of the most significant bloodborne pathogens include hepatitis B virus, and human immunodeficiency virus. Other bloodborne diseases include hepatitis C, delta hepatitis, syphilis, and malaria.

EXPOSURE LIMITS

There are no exposure limits for this occupational category.

TARGET ORGAN(S) AND POTENTIAL HEALTH EFFECTS

The target organs and potential health effects will depend upon the hazards to which the employee is exposed (i.e. bloodborne diseases). These bloodborne pathogens may be transmitted from the infected individual to other individuals by blood or certain other body fluids. Hepatitis means "inflammation of the liver," and can be caused by a number of agents or conditions including drugs, toxins, autoimmune disease, and infectious agents including viruses. The most common causes of hepatitis are viruses. Acquired Immunodeficiency Syndrome (AIDS) or human immunodeficiency virus type 1 (HIV-1) can be transmitted through occupational exposure to blood or other potentially infectious materials.

CRITERIA FOR ENTRY INTO MEDICAL SURVEILLANCE PROGRAM

There are no mandatory criteria for entrance into medical surveillance programs for individuals exposed to blood and body fluids. However, the EHS must offer the HBV vaccine unless already immune or vaccine contraindicated. If exposed specific post-exposure monitoring for employee and source must be administered refer to 29 CFR 1910.1030.

SURVEILLANCE FREQUENCY

No pre-placement evaluations are required excepted the company must offer Hepatitis B (HBV) vaccine unless already immune or vaccine contraindicated.

Emergency/exposure examination and tests include specific post-exposure monitoring for employee and source (refer to CFR 29 1910.103(f)).

MEDICAL AND OCCUPATIONAL HISTORY

The medical and occupational history should concentrate on those conditions or exposures that may place the worker at increased risk for infection. The following specific areas should be emphasized (refer to Appendix B).

History of specific post-exposure to blood borne pathogens and monitoring for employee and sources.

A hepatitis B vaccination form, should be completed and in the worker's medical record if worker declines to receive the hepatitis B vaccination series.

PHYSICAL EXAMINATION

There are no physical examination requirements for bloodborne pathogens.

LABORATORY

A post-exposure incident test, which follows the U.S. Public Health Service post-exposure protocols, may be required.

Table 4-1: Bloodborne Pathogens

Requirements For Bloodborne Pathogens 1910.1030(f)	
Pre-placement exam	No – must offer Hepatitis B (HBV) vaccine unless already immune or vaccine contraindicated
Periodic exam	No
Emergency/exposure Examination and Tests	Specific post-exposure monitoring for employee and source; HBV vaccine; see standard.
Termination exam	No
Examination includes special emphasis on these body systems	No
Work and medical history	No
Chest x-ray	No
Pulmonary function test (PFT)	No
Other required tests	Yes-post-exposure incident; follow US Public Health Service(USPHS) post-exposure protocols
Evaluation of ability to wear A respirator	No
Additional Tests if deemed necessary	Yes-for post-exposure incident; follow USPHS post-exposure protocols
Written medical opinion	Yes-licensed health care professional to employer; employer to employee
Employee counseling re: exam results, Conditions of increased risk	Yes-by licensed health care professional; counseling re: HBV vaccine and post-exposure follow-up; see standard
Medical removal plan	No

Chapter 5: Respiratory Protection

HAZARD DESCRIPTION

When respirators are worn in toxic atmospheres, the individual's body burden may be evaluated using appropriate laboratory tests. These may include urine, blood, or fecal analysis and other techniques to determine the intake and excretion of toxic substances. The findings of these tests, when correlated with other exposure data, such as air sampling data for wearers of such equipment, can serve as an indication of the effectiveness of the program. Positive evidence of exposure must be followed up with appropriate surveillance of work area conditions to determine if there is any relationship to inadequate respiratory protection or a need for additional engineering controls

Respirators are an effective method of protection against designated hazards when properly selected and worn. Respirator use is encouraged, even when exposures are below the exposure limit, to provide an additional level of comfort and protection for workers. However, if a respirator is used improperly or not kept clean, the respirator itself can become a hazard to the worker. Sometimes, workers may wear respirators to avoid exposures to hazards, even if the amount of hazardous substance does not exceed the limits set by OSHA standards. If your employer provides respirators for your voluntary use, or if you provide your own respirator, you need to take certain precautions to be sure that the respirator itself does not present a hazard.

EXPOSURE LIMITS

The exposure limits for the worker depends on the hazardous materials in the worker's environment.

CRITERIA FOR ENTRY INTO THE MEDICAL SURVEILLANCE PROGRAM

Given the increased resistance that respirators place on the heart/lungs, EHS is required to send their potential respirator users to a medical physician.

The physician screens each potential respirator user for ability to safely (psychologically and physically) wear a respirator, by taking into consideration the medical signs, symptoms and conditions.

This evaluation includes:

1. Having the employee complete a confidential medical questionnaire (designed by OSHA);

2. Obtaining additional medical history (as necessary);

3. Performing a pulmonary function test, PFT (spirometry); and

4. (Based on the information obtained) potentially a chest x-ray

The physician then provides EHS with a "Medical Fitness Qualification Form" OSHA requires that this medical evaluation be performed only once, unless the user's medical condition changes.

- In order to alert employees to the possibility that a repeat medical evaluation may be necessary, EHS provides each employee with a "Medical Fitness Status Form" to be completed at his/her annual EH&S "Fit Test".

- This "Medical Fitness Status Form" lists the medical signs/symptoms/conditions which can limit safe use of respirators (provided in the company's Respirator Safety Program and asks each user to review the list and respond whether he/she has developed any of these symptoms since their last medical respirator evaluation. If "yes", EH&S notifies the employee's supervisor to schedule a follow-up medical evaluation.

PHYSICAL EXAMINATION

Evaluation questionnaire or exam and follow-up exam when required every one to three years depending on medical condition (refer to Appendix E).

Table 5-1: Requirements For Respiratory Protection

Requirements For Respiratory Protection 1910.134(e)/1926.103	
Pre-placement exam	Evaluation questionnaire or exam; follow-up exam when required.
Periodic exam	Yes—1-3 years depending on Medical Condition
Emergency/exposure Examination and Tests	No
Termination exam	No
Examination includes special emphasis on these body systems	Yes—see standard, Appendix C
Work and medical history	Yes—see standard, Appendix C
Chest x-ray	As determined by physician or other licensed health care professional
Pulmonary function test (PFT)	As determined by physician or other licensed health care professional
Other required tests	As determined by physician or other licensed health care professional
Evaluation of ability to wear A respirator	Yes
Additional Tests if deemed necessary	Yes
Written medical opinion	Yes-- licensed health care professional to employer; employer to employee
Employee counseling re: exam results, Conditions of increased risk	Yes—by physician or other licensed health care professional
Medical removal plan	No

Chapter 6: Noise

Noise, or unwanted sound, is one of the most pervasive occupational health problems. It is a by-product of many industrial processes. Sound consists of pressure changes in a medium (usually air), caused by vibration or turbulence. These pressure changes produce waves emanating away from the turbulent or vibrating source.

HAZARDOUS DESCRIPTION

Exposure to high levels of noise causes hearing loss and may cause other harmful health effects as well. The extent of damage depends primarily on the intensity of the noise and the duration of the exposure. Noise-induced hearing loss can be temporary or permanent. Temporary hearing loss results from short-term exposures to noise, with normal hearing returning after a period of rest. Generally, prolonged exposure to high noise levels over a period of time gradually causes permanent damage.

EXPOSURE LIMITS

Any employee whose exposure to noise levels equal or exceed an 8-hour time weighted average.

The employer shall establish and maintain an audiometric testing program as proved in 29 CFR 1910.95 by making audiometric testing available to all employees whose exposures equal or exceed an 8-hour time-weighted average of 85 decibels.

TARGET ORGAN(S) AND POTENTIAL HEALTH EFFECTS

Noise above 85 decibels effect the cochlea which leads to hearing loss.

CRITERIA FOR ENTRY INTO MEDICAL SURVEILLANCE PROGRAM

Within six months of an employee's first exposure at or above the action level, the employer shall establish a valid baseline audiogram against which subsequent audiograms can be compared (1910.95(g)(5)(i)).

SURVEILLANCE FREQUENCY

At least annually after obtaining the baseline audiogram, the employer shall obtain a new audiogram for each employee exposed at or above an eight-hour time-weighted average of 85 decibels (1910.95(g)(6)).

Each employee's annual audiogram shall be compared to that employee's baseline audiogram to determine if the audiogram is valid and if a standard threshold shift. This comparison may be done by a technician (1910.95(g)(7)(ii)).

If the annual audiogram shows that an employee has suffered a standard threshold shift, the employer may obtain a retest within 30 days and consider the results of the retest as the annual audiogram (1910.95(g)(7)(ii)).

The audiologist, otolaryngologist, or physician shall review problem audiograms and shall determine whether there is a need for further evaluation (1910.95(g)(7)(iii)).

FOLLOW-UP PROCEDURE

If a comparison of the annual audiogram to the baseline audiogram indicates a standard threshold shift has occurred, the employee shall be informed of this fact in writing, within 21 days of the determination (1910.95(g)(8)(i)).

Unless a physician determines that the standard threshold shift is not work related or aggravated by occupational noise exposure, the employer shall ensure that the following steps are taken when a standard threshold shift occurs (1910.95(g)(8)(ii)–(g)(8)(ii)(D)):

(A) Employees not using hearing protectors shall be fitted with hearing protectors, trained in their use and care, and required to use them.

(B) Employees already using hearing protectors shall be refitted and retrained in the use of hearing protectors and provided with hearing protectors offering greater attenuation if necessary.

(C) The employee shall be referred for a clinical audiological evaluation or an otological examination, as appropriate, if additional testing is necessary or if the employer suspects that a medical pathology of the ear is caused or aggravated by the wearing of hearing protectors.

(D) The employee is informed of the need for an otological examination if a medical pathology of the ear that is unrelated to the use of hearing protectors is suspected

MEDICAL AND OCCUPATIONAL HISTORY

The medical and occupational history should concentrate on those conditions or exposure that may place the workers at increased risk for hearing loss.

PHYSICAL EXAMINATION

A pre-placement examination is not required, however, an audiometric testing examination is required.

TERMINATION EXAMINATION

A termination audiometric examination is required at the end of the worker's employment.

Table 6-1: Requirements for Noise

Requirements For Noise 1910.95(g)/1926.52	
Pre-placement exam	Audiometric testing required. No physical exam.
Periodic exam	Audiometric testing required. No physical exam.
Emergency/exposure Examination and Tests	No
Termination exam	Audiometric testing required. No physical exam
Examination includes special emphasis on these body systems	No
Work and medical history	No
Chest x-ray	No
Pulmonary function test (PFT)	No
Other required tests	Initial and annual audiometric testing; see standard re:specific qualifications for the test administrator
Evaluation of ability to wear A respirator	No
Additional Tests if deemed necessary	Yes
Written medical opinion	No
Employee counseling re: exam results, Conditions of increased risk	Yes—if standard threshold shift or suspected ear pathology
Medical removal plan	No

Chapter 7: Pesticides (Organophosphate And Carbamate) Applicators

Organophosphate and carbamate pesticides are routinely used in a variety of pest control applications. These substances are grouped together because of a common mode of toxic action—the inhibition of the enzyme cholinesterase. Organophosphates, as a class, generally bind to the enzyme irreversibly while carbamates tend to bind reversibly. Human toxicity from these compounds can vary widely. Nearly all are readily absorbed from dermal contact, inhalation, and ingestion, making it essential for medical personnel to evaluate the exposure conditions and work practices of the applicators to assess the exposure hazards from multiple routes. Examples of compounds included in this category are: organophosphate pesticides—Dichlorvos (CAS # 62-73-7); Diazinon (CAS# 333-41-5); Chlorpyrifos (CAS# 2921-88-2); Malathion (CAS#121-75-5); and carbamate pesticides—Carbaryl (CAS# 63-25-2); Thiram (CAS#137-26-8); Propoxur (CAS#114-26-1); Ficam (CAS# 22781-23-1).

HAZARDOUS DESCRIPTION

Organophosphates and carbamates exert their toxic effects by inhibiting cholinesterase in synapses. In acute exposures, initial hyperstimulation is followed by blockage of the affected synapses. Acute symptoms are excessive bronchial secretions, salivation, respiratory distress, incontinence, pinpoint pupils, fasiculations, abdominal cramps, tremors, cyanosis, and coma.

EXPOSURE LIMITS

Many organophosphate and carbamate pesticides have exposure limits (PEL) that are included in the OSHA Z-table. Exposure limits for these pesticides carry a skin designation to emphasize that they can be absorbed through the skin.

TARGET ORGANS(S) AND POTENTIAL HEALTH EFFECTS

The major target organs for organophosphate and carbamate pesticides are the peripheral and central nervous systems.

CRITERIA FOR ENTRY IN MEDICAL SURVEILLANCE PROGRAM

Personnel should be entered into medical surveillance if they are: exposed to airborne concentrations above the action level for 30 or more days per year; at significant risk of absorption from dermal exposure or ingestion; or performing an operation in an area where a worker has experienced toxicity related to pesticide exposure and exposure controls have not been in place long enough to assess their effectiveness. In addition, if a workplace survey identifies significant potential for dermal absorption or ingestion, appropriate hazard controls and work practice changes should be recommended. Medical surveillance may be used in these cases as an adjunct to industrial hygiene monitoring to determine if hazard controls are working. Medical monitoring should not be used as a substitute for industrial hygiene surveys.

SURVEILLANCE FREQUENCY

Workers identified for medical surveillance should receive pre-placement, periodic, and termination of exposure examinations. Cholinesterase determinations will be done during the maximum usage period of the pesticide application season. At locations where organophosphate pesticides are used year-round, the worker should receive at least quarterly cholinesterase determinations. All workers should be examined following any emergency over exposure.

Note: Because reduced cholinesterase activity can be transient, medical surveillance should be performed during the period of time workers are engaging in operations using organophosphate and carbamate pesticides. Sampling workers at times when they are not exposed is of no value and may mislead workers into believing work practices and applications operations are not producing significant exposures.

MEDICAL AND OCCUPATIONAL HISTORY

At each periodic evaluation, the workers history of use and exposure to pesticides and use of personal protective equipment should be reviewed and updated. A general medical history, along with a specific review of systems emphasizing symptoms of organophosphate/carbamate pesticide toxicity, i.e. headache, salivation, muscle twitching, should be updated or obtained at each evaluation (refer to Appendix B).

PHYSICAL EXAMINATION

When acute toxicity is suspected, the worker should have a complete neurological exam (including evaluation of pupillary size and reactivity and observation for muscle fasiculations and tremor), auscultation of the chest for wheezing, and inspection for cyanosis.

Routine periodic examinations during the pesticide use season may be limited to the medical and occupational history and cholinesterase testing. Physical examinations for signs of mild exposures are not recommended.

LABORATORY

Serum (or plasma) and red blood cell (RBC) cholinesterase baseline levels should be done at preplacement or before exposure. This baseline value should be the average of two or more tests taken at least 72 hours, but not more than 14 days apart, and analyzed at the same laboratory. If two tests are done and the difference between them exceeds 15%, a third baseline test should be performed. The average of the two closest values should be considered the true baseline value. All baseline tests should be taken when the worker has had no exposure to cholinesterase inhibitors for at least 30 days. Since the interpretation of cholinesterase levels may be difficult, the following guidance is provided under the guidelines.[12]

Serum (or plasma) cholinesterase has a relatively short half-life whereas RBC cholinesterase has the same half-life as red blood cells (about 120 days). These two enzymes are structurally distinct and are inhibited differently by the various organophosphate and carbamate pesticides. For example, diazinon inhibits serum cholinesterase to a much greater extent than RBC cholinesterase under pesticides studied in man[13]. Whereas, carbaryl inhibits both serum and RBC cholinesterase. The normal ranges for serum and RBC cholinesterase determinations are wide with marked interindividual variability and variability if different analytical methods or laboratories are used. For this reason, baseline pre-exposure measurements done by the same methodology, and preferably by the same laboratory are extremely important. Individuals should be compared against their baseline levels rather than the "normal" range. A reduction in serum cholinesterase activity to 60% of baseline may occur before any symptoms appear and a drop to 20% of baseline activity is required before serious neuromuscular symptoms become apparent. A variety of medical conditions can depress cholinesterase activity.

A drop in plasma or RBC cholinesterase levels to 80% of a worker's baseline or lower indicates the need for retesting. If the low value is confirmed, the employer should investigate the workplace for faulty work practices and take corrective measures. A drop in RBC cholinesterase level to 70% of baseline or lower, or a drop in plasma cholinesterase level to 60% of baseline or lower, indicates a need for immediate removal of the worker from all exposure to cholinesterase inhibitors until both parameters return to within 80% of the preexposure baseline or higher under the guidelines.[12]

In some cases, if exposure to a specific pesticide is suspected, tests for either the chemical or a metabolic product are available. Measurement of urinary organic phosphates is a helpful adjunct to cholinesterase determinations in workers suspected of significant organophosphate exposure. Total urinary organic phosphates in excess of 0.1 mg/L are evidence of significant exposure to organophosphate insecticides. Determination of urinary 1-naphthol is helpful in evaluating workers with suspected exposures to carbaryl. Urinary 1-naphthol levels, measured by colorimetry, greater than 4 mg/L represent significant exposures to carbaryl under 29 U.S.C. 651 et seq and the guidelines.[14, 15]

OTHER ELEMENTS

Removal from exposure if medically indicated by the drop in plasma or RBC cholinesterase levels.

If respirators are used to protect workers from this hazard, the requirements of the companies Respiratory Safety Program and 29 CFR 1910.134 should be applied to assess the worker's ability to safely use the respirator.

Workers should receive education on the routes of exposure, and the particular importance of dermal exposure; the importance of hand washing and personal hygiene to minimize exposure; and of the symptoms that could represent absorption.

A health care practitioner's written opinion indicating that the worker is qualified for work with organophosphate or carbamate pesticides may be used if desired.

Table 7-1: Requirements for organophosphate and Carbamate Pesticides Applicators

Requirements For organophosphate and Carbamate Pesticides Applicators	
Pre-placement exam	Yes
Periodic exam	Yes – Annual Exam
Emergency/exposure Examination and Tests	Yes
Termination exam	Yes
Examination includes special emphasis on these body systems	Blood, respiratory, heart, kidney
Work and medical history	Yes
Chest x-ray	As determined by a physician or other licensed health care professional
Pulmonary function test (PFT)	Yes – if using a respiratory
Other required tests	Cholinesterase baseline blood drawn prior to exposure.
Evaluation of ability to wear A respirator	Yes
Additional Tests if deemed necessary	Yes
Written medical opinion	Yes
Employee counseling re: exam results, Conditions of increased risk	Yes – by physician or other licensed health care professional.
Medical removal plan	No

Chapter 8: Aerial Work Platform

CRITERIA FOR ENTRY INTO THE MEDICAL SURVEILLANCE PROGRAM

A medical screening questionnaire is required for new and renewal aerial work platform operators. The questionnaire will be completed by the employee and mailed confidentially to the company's occupational health care provider.

EXCEPTION

Employees who are in the medical surveillance program for other reasons (such as respirator wearers) will not receive a questionnaire since they have already had a physical exam at the clinic. When they are due for the annual exam, the supervisor will receive the medical request form for review and approval.

SURVEILLANCE FREQUENCY

A questionnaire is required at the time of the employee's initial and renewal their aerial work platform permit.

MEDICAL AND OCCUPATIONAL HISTORY

The medical and occupational history should concentrate on those conditions that may place the worker at increased risk for harm (refer to Appendix F).

PHYSICAL EXAMINATION

A physician may request a pre-physical examination for the employee, if the questionnaire red flags any condition that should be further evaluated before making a final determination. Upon completion of the medical evaluation, the occupational health care provider will send a Determination Form to the Departmental Medical Surveillance contact person and EHS. The Office of Environmental Health and Safety will keep the Determination Forms on record and track the medical screening process.

Table 8-1: Requirements For Aerial Platform Operators

Requirements For Aerial Work Platform Operators	
Pre-placement exam	Yes – If a physician determines to be necessary. **A medical questionnaire is required to be given**
Periodic exam	Renewal of permit or every three years.
Emergency/exposure Examination and Tests	No
Termination exam	No
Examination includes special emphasis on these body systems	As determine by a physician or other licensed health care professional.
Work and medical history	Yes
Chest x-ray	No
Pulmonary function test (PFT)	Yes, if using a respiratory or determined by a physician or other licensed health care professional
Other required tests	As determine by a physician or other licensed health care professional.
Evaluation of ability to wear A respirator	Yes, if using a respiratory or determined by a physician or other licensed health care professional
Additional Tests if deemed necessary	As determine by a physician or other licensed health care professional.
Written medical opinion	Yes
Employee counseling re: exam results, Conditions of increased risk	No
Medical removal plan	No

Chapter 9: Formaldehyde Exposure

HAZARD DESCRIPTION

The occupational health hazards of formaldehyde are primarily due to its toxic effects after inhalation, after direct contact with the skin or eyes by formaldehyde in liquid or vapor form, and after ingestion.

ACUTE EFFECTS OF EXPOSURE

Inhalation (breathing): Formaldehyde is highly irritating to the upper airways. The concentration of formaldehyde that is immediately dangerous to life and health is 100 ppm. Concentrations above 50 ppm can cause severe pulmonary reactions within minutes. These include pulmonary edema, pneumonia, and bronchial irritation which can result in death. Concentrations above 5 ppm readily cause lower airway irritation characterized by cough, chest tightness and wheezing. There is some controversy regarding whether formaldehyde gas is a pulmonary sensitizer which can cause occupational asthma in a previously normal individual. Formaldehyde can produce symptoms of bronchial asthma in humans. The mechanism may be either sensitization of the individual by exposure to formaldehyde or direct irritation by formaldehyde in persons with pre-existing asthma. Upper airway irritation is the most common respiratory effect reported by workers and can occur over a wide range of concentrations, most frequently above 1 ppm. However, airway irritation has occurred in some workers with exposures to formaldehyde as low as 0.1 ppm. Symptoms of upper airway irritation include dry or sore throat, itching and burning sensations of the nose, and nasal congestion. Tolerance to this level of exposure may develop within 1-2 hours. This tolerance can permit workers remaining in an environment of gradually increasing formaldehyde concentrations to be unaware of their increasingly hazardous exposure.

Eye contact: Concentrations of formaldehyde between 0.05 ppm and 0.5 ppm produce a sensation of irritation in the eyes with burning, itching, redness, and tearing. Increased rate of blinking and eye closure generally protects the eye from damage at these low levels, but these protective mechanisms may interfere with some workers' work abilities. Tolerance can occur in workers continuously exposed to concentrations of formaldehyde in this range. Accidental splash injuries of human eyes to aqueous solutions of formaldehyde (formalin) have resulted in a wide range of ocular injuries including corneal opacities and blindness. The severity of the reactions has been directly dependent on the concentration of formaldehyde in solution and the amount of time lapsed before emergency and medical intervention.

Skin contact: Exposure to formaldehyde solutions can cause irritation of the skin and allergic contact dermatitis. These skin diseases and disorders can occur at levels well below those encountered by many formaldehyde workers. Symptoms include erythema, edema, and vesiculation or hives. Exposure to liquid formalin or formaldehyde vapor can provoke skin reactions in sensitized individuals even when airborne concentrations of formaldehyde are well below 1 ppm.

Ingestion: Ingestion of as little as 30 ml of a 37 percent solution of formaldehyde (formalin) can result in death. Gastrointestinal toxicity after ingestion is most severe in the stomach and results in symptoms which can include nausea, vomiting, and severe abdominal pain. Diverse damage to other organ systems including the liver, kidney, spleen, pancreas, brain, and central nervous systems can occur from the acute response to ingestion of formaldehyde.

CHRONIC EFFECTS OF EXPOSURE

Long term exposure to formaldehyde has been shown to be associated with an increased risk of cancer of the nose and accessory sinuses, nasopharyngeal and oropharyngeal cancer, and lung cancer in humans. Animal experiments provide conclusive evidence of a causal relationship between nasal cancer in rats and formaldehyde exposure. Concordant evidence of carcinogenicity includes DNA binding, genotoxicity in short-term tests, and cytotoxic changes in the cells of the target organ suggesting both preneoplastic changes and a dose-rate effect. Formaldehyde is a complete carcinogen and appears to exert an effect on at least two stages of the carcinogenic process.

EXPOSURE LIMITS

The employer shall institute medical surveillance programs for all employees exposed to formaldehyde at concentrations at or exceeding the action level or exceeding the short-term exposure limit (STEL) (1910.1048(l)(1)(i)).

The employer shall assure that no employee is exposed to an airborne concentration of formaldehyde which exceeds 0.75 parts formaldehyde per million parts of air (0.75 ppm) as an 8-hour time weight average (TWA) (1910.1048(c)(1)).

The employer shall assure that no employee is exposed to an airborne concentration of formaldehyde which exceeds two parts formaldehyde per million parts of air (2 ppm) as a 15-minute STEL (1910.1048(c)(2)).

The employer shall make medical surveillance available for employees who develop signs and symptoms of overexposure to formaldehyde and for all employees exposed to formaldehyde in emergencies. When determining whether an employee may be experiencing signs and symptoms of possible overexposure to formaldehyde, the employer may rely on the evidence that signs and symptoms associated with formaldehyde exposure will occur only in exceptional circumstances when airborne exposure is less than 0.1 ppm and when formaldehyde is present in material in concentrations less than 0.1 percent (1910.1048(l)(1)(ii)).

CRITERIA FOR ENTRY INTO THE MEDICAL SURVEILLANCE PROGRAM

The program consists of screening formaldehyde-exposed employees, with follow-up medical examinations in those instances when the physician feels it necessary. As a minimum, the screening consists of the administration of a questionnaire, which must include a work history, a smoking history, and elicits information on a variety of medical conditions associated with formaldehyde exposure. These conditions include eye, nose, or throat irritation, chronic airway problems or hyperactive airway disease, allergic skin conditions or dermatitis, and upper and lower respiratory problems.

A medical disease questionnaire will be given to the employee such as Appendix G. The company will "make the following medical surveillance available to employees prior to assignment to a job where formaldehyde exposure is at or above the action level or above the STEL and annually thereafter. The employer shall also make the following medical surveillance available promptly upon determining that an employee is experiencing signs and symptoms indicative of possible overexposure to formaldehyde " (1910.1048(l)(3)).

SURVEILLANCE FREQUENCY

All employees exposed to formaldehyde at or above the action Level or STEL must be screened annually, by means of a medical questionnaire. In addition, employees exposed to formaldehyde must be screened with the questionnaire if they develop signs or symptoms of possible formaldehyde-related illness. If the responsible physician, upon evaluating the questionnaire, determines that a medical examination is necessary, the employee must be examined, and given any tests which the physician feels are appropriate.

MEDICAL AND OCCUPATIONAL HISTORY

Formaldehyde can cause allergic sensitization and cancer. One of the goals of the work history should be to elicit information on any prior or additional exposure to formaldehyde in either the occupational or the non-occupational setting.

Respiratory History

As noted above, formaldehyde has recognized properties as an airway irritant and has been reported by some authors as a cause of occupational asthma. In addition, formaldehyde has been associated with cancer of the entire respiratory system of humans. For these reasons, it is appropriate to include a comprehensive review of the respiratory system in the medical history. Components of this history might include questions regarding dyspnea on exertion, shortness of breath, chronic airway complaints, hyperreactive airway disease, rhinitis, bronchitis, bronchiolitis, asthma, emphysema, respiratory allergic reaction, or other preexisting pulmonary disease.

In addition, generalized airway hypersensitivity can result from exposures to a single sensitizing agent. The examiner should, therefore, elicit any prior history of exposure to pulmonary irritants, and any short- or long-term effects of that exposure.

Smoking is known to decrease mucociliary clearance of materials deposited during respiration in the nose and upper airways. This may increase a worker's exposure to inhaled materials such as formaldehyde vapor. In addition, smoking is a potential confounding factor in the investigation of any chronic respiratory disease, including cancer. For these reasons, a complete smoking history should be obtained.

Skin Disorders

Because of the dermal irritant and sensitizing effects of formaldehyde, a history of skin disorders should be obtained. Such a history might include the existence of skin irritation, previously documented skin sensitivity, and other dermatologic disorders. Previous exposure to formaldehyde and other dermal sensitizers should be recorded.

History Of Atopic Or Allergic Diseases

Since formaldehyde can cause allergic sensitization of the skin and airways, it might be useful to identify individuals with prior allergen sensitization. A history of atopic disease and allergies to formaldehyde or any other substances should also be obtained. It is not definitely known at this time whether atopic diseases and allergies to formaldehyde or any other substances should also be obtained. Also it is not definitely known at this time whether atopic individuals have a greater propensity to develop formaldehyde sensitivity than the general population, but identification of these individuals may be useful for ongoing surveillance.

PHYSICAL EXAMINATION

Employer Obligations

The employer is required to provide the physician with the following information: A copy of this standard and 29 CFR 1910.1048 Appendices A, C, D, and E; a description of the affected employee's duties as they relate to his or her exposure concentration; an estimate of the employee's exposure including duration (e.g. 15 hr/wk, three 8-hour shifts, full-time); a description of any personal protective equipment, including respirators, used by the employee; and the results of any previous medical determinations for the affected employee related to formaldehyde exposure to the extent that this information is within the employer's control (1910.1048(l)(6)-(l)(6)(vi).

Examination by a Physician

All medical procedures, including administration of medical disease questionnaires, shall be performed by or under the supervision of a licensed physician and shall be provided without cost to the employee, without loss of pay, and at a reasonable time and place (1910.1048(l)(2)).

A determination by the physician, based on evaluation of the medical disease questionnaire, of whether a medical examination is necessary for employees not required to wear respirators to reduce exposure to formaldehyde (1910.1048 (l)(3)(ii)).

Medical examinations shall be given to any employee who the physician feels, based on information in the medical disease questionnaire, may be at increased risk from exposure to formaldehyde and at the time of initial assignment and at least annually thereafter to all employees required to wear a respirator to reduce exposure to formaldehyde. The medical examination shall include:

A physical examination with emphasis on evidence of irritation or sensitization of the skin and respiratory system, shortness of breath, or irritation of the eyes (1910.1048 (l)(4)–(l)(4)(i)).

Emergency Exposure Examination

The examination of workers exposed in an emergency should be directed at the organ systems most likely to be affected. Much of the content of the examination will be similar to the periodic examination unless the patient has received a severe acute exposure requiring immediate attention to prevent serious consequences. If a severe overexposure requiring medical intervention or hospitalization has occurred, the physician must be alert to the possibility of delayed symptoms. Follow-up nonroutine examinations may be necessary to assure the patient's well being.

Physician Written Statement

For each examination required under this standard, the employer shall obtain a written opinion from the examining physician. This written opinion shall contain the results of the medical examination except that it shall not reveal specific findings or diagnoses unrelated to occupational exposure to formaldehyde. The written opinion shall include (1910.1048(l)(7)(i)(A)–(l)(7)(i)(C)):

(A) The physician's opinion as to whether the employee has any medical condition that would place the employee at an increased risk of material impairment of health from exposure to formaldehyde;

(B) Any recommended limitations on the employee's exposure or changes in the use of personal protective equipment, including respirators;

(C) A statement that the employee has been informed by the physician of any medical conditions which would be aggravated by exposure to formaldehyde, whether these conditions may have resulted from past formaldehyde exposure or from exposure in an emergency, and whether there is a need for further examination or treatment.

The employer shall provide for retention of the results of the medical examination and tests conducted by the physician (1910.1048(l)(7)(ii)).

The employer shall provide a copy of the physician's written opinion to the affected employee within 15 days of its receipt (1910.1048(l)(7)(iii)).

Medical Removal or Restriction

The provisions of paragraph 1910.1048 (l)(8) apply when an employee reports significant irritation of the mucosa of the eyes or of the upper airways, respiratory sensitization, dermal irritation, or dermal sensitization attributed to workplace formaldehyde exposure. Medical removal provisions do not apply in the case of dermal irritation or dermal sensitization when the product suspected of causing the dermal condition contains less than 0.05 percent formaldehyde (1910.1048(l)(8)(i)).

An employee's report of signs or symptoms of possible overexposure to formaldehyde shall be evaluated by a physician selected by the employer pursuant to paragraph (l)(3). If the physician determines that a medical examination is not necessary under paragraph (l)(3)(ii), there shall be a two-week evaluation and remediation period to permit the employer to ascertain whether the signs or symptoms subside untreated or with the use of creams, gloves, first aid treatment or personal protective equipment. Industrial hygiene measures that limit the employee's exposure to formaldehyde may also be implemented during this period. The employee shall be referred immediately to a physician prior to expiration of the two-week period if the signs or symptoms worsen. Earnings, seniority and benefits may not be altered during the two-week period by virtue of the report (1910.1048(l)(8)(ii)).

If the signs or symptoms have not subsided or been remedied by the end of the two-week period, or earlier if signs or symptoms warrant, the employee shall be examined by a physician selected by the employer. The physician shall presume, absent contrary evidence, that observed dermal irritation or dermal sensitization is not attributable to formaldehyde when products to which the affected employee is exposed contain less than 0.1 percent formaldehyde (1910.1048(l)(8)(iii)).

Medical examinations shall be conducted in compliance with the requirements of paragraph (l)(5)(i) and (ii). Additional guidelines for conducting medical exams are contained in Appendix C (1910.1048(l)(8)(iv)).

If the physician finds that significant irritation of the mucosa of the eyes or of the upper airways, respiratory sensitization, dermal irritation, or dermal sensitization result from workplace formaldehyde exposure and recommends restrictions or removal, the employer shall promptly comply with the restrictions or recommendation of removal. In the event of a recommendation of removal, the employer shall remove the affected employee from the current formaldehyde exposure and if possible, transfer the employee to work having no or significantly less exposure to formaldehyde (1910.1048(l)(8)(v)).

When an employee is removed pursuant to paragraph (l)(8)(v), the employer shall transfer the employee to comparable work for which the employee is qualified or can be trained in a short period (up to 6 months), where the formaldehyde exposures are as low as possible, but not higher than the action level. The employer shall maintain the employee's current earnings, seniority, and other benefits. If there is no such work available, the employer shall maintain the employee's current earnings, seniority and other benefits until such work becomes available, until the employee is determined to be unable to return to workplace formaldehyde exposure, until the employee is determined to be able to return to the original job status, or for six months, whichever comes first (1910.1048(l)(8)(vi)).

The employer shall arrange for a follow-up medical examination to take place within six months after the employee is removed pursuant to this paragraph. This examination shall determine if the employee can return to the original job status, or if the removal is to be permanent. The physician shall make a decision within six months of the date the employee was removed as to whether the employee can be returned to the original job status, or if the removal is to be permanent (1910.1048(l)(8)(vii)).

An employer's obligation to provide earnings, seniority and other benefits to a removed employee may be reduced to the extent that the employee receives compensation for earnings lost during the period of removal either from a publicly or employer-funded compensation program or from employment with another employer made possible by virtue of the employee's removal (1910.1048(l)(8)(viii)).

In making determinations of the formaldehyde content of materials under this paragraph the employer may rely on objective data (1910.1048(l)(8)(ix)).

LABORATORY

The physician may deem it necessary to perform other medical examinations or tests as indicated. The standard provides a mechanism whereby these additional investigations are covered under the standard for occupational exposure to formaldehyde.

Table 9-1: Requirements For Formaldehyde

Requirements For Formaldehyde 1910.1048(l)/1926.1148	
Pre-placement exam	Yes – emphasis on eye irritation irritation/sensitization of skin or respiratory system or shortness of breath.
Periodic exam	Yes
Emergency/exposure Examination and Tests	Yes
Termination exam	No
Examination includes special emphasis on these body systems	Evidence of irritation or sensitization of skin, respiratory system, eyes; shortness of breath.
Work and medical history	Required for all exams; questionnaire required; see standard Appendix D
Chest x-ray	No
Pulmonary function test (PFT)	FVC, FEV, FEF should be evaluated if respiratory protection is used
Other required tests	No
Evaluation of ability to wear a respirator	Yes
Additional Tests if deemed necessary	Yes
Written medical opinion	Yes—physician to employer; employer to employee
Employee counseling re: exam results, Conditions of increased risk	Yes—by physician; includes information on whether medical conditions were caused by past exposures or emergency exposures.
Medical removal plan	Yes

Chapter 10: Heat Stress For Extremely Hot Environments

HAZARD DESCRIPTION

Work operations involving high air temperatures, radiant heat sources, high humidity, direct physical contact with hot objects, or strenuous physical activities have a high potential for inducing heat stress in employees engaged in such operations. These activities are often conducted in the following locations: the steam tunnels; sections of the Central Heating Plant; pipe chases; some mechanical rooms; outdoor construction activities; particularly on roofs; and outdoor construction activities that require the use of protective clothing.

Although no one questions that there is a relation between heat stress and occupational accidents, it is difficult to predict who will be affected and when. Two people can work at the same job, under the same conditions, and while the heat will affect one, the other will not. Age, weight, degree of physical fitness, degree of acclimatization, metabolism, use of alcohol or drugs and a variety of medical conditions all affect a person's sensitivity to heat. Even the type of clothing worn must be considered. In addition, the measurement of a hot environment involves more than just measuring the ambient air temperature—radiant heat, air movement, and relative humidity are all factors that must be determined.

The risk of heat-induced illnesses and injuries may be increased and productivity reduced in situations when the total heat load exceeds the capacities of the body to maintain normal body functions. This program is to assist supervisors in eliminating or reducing those risk factors.

Heat Stroke

Heat stroke occurs when the body's system of temperature regulation fails and body temperature rises to critical levels. This condition is caused by a combination of highly variable factors, and its occurrence is difficult to predict.

Heat stroke is a medical emergency. The primary signs and symptoms of heat stroke are confusion; irrational behavior; loss of consciousness; convulsions; a lack of sweating (usually); hot, dry skin; and an abnormally high body temperature, e.g., a rectal temperature of 41 degrees C (105.8 degrees F). If body temperature is too high, it causes death. The elevated metabolic temperatures caused by a combination of workload and environmental heat load, both of which contribute to heat stroke, are also highly variable and difficult to predict.

If a worker shows signs of possible heat stroke, professional medical treatment should be obtained immediately. The worker should be placed in a shady area and the outer clothing should be removed. The worker's skin should be wetted and air movement around the worker should be increased to improve evaporative cooling until professional methods of cooling are initiated and the seriousness of the condition can be assessed. Fluids should be replaced as soon as possible. The medical outcome of an episode of heat stroke depends on the victim's physical fitness and the timing and effectiveness of first aid treatment.

Regardless of the worker's protests, no employee suspected of being ill from heat stroke should be sent home or left unattended unless a physician has specifically approved such an order.

Heat Exhaustion

The signs and symptoms of heat exhaustion are headache, nausea, vertigo, weakness, thirst, and giddiness. Fortunately, this condition responds readily to prompt treatment.

Heat exhaustion should not be dismissed lightly, however, for several reasons. One is that the fainting associated with heat exhaustion can be dangerous because the victim may be operating machinery or controlling an operation that should not be left unattended; moreover, the victim may be injured when he or she faints. Also, the signs and symptoms seen in heat exhaustion are similar to those of heat stroke, a medical emergency.

Workers suffering from heat exhaustion should be removed from the hot environment and given fluid replacement. They should also be encouraged to get adequate rest.

Heat Cramps

Performing hard physical labor in a hot environment usually causes heat cramps. These cramps have been attributed to an electrolyte imbalance caused by sweating. It is important to understand that cramps can be caused by both too much and too little salt.

Cramps appear to be caused by the lack of water replenishment. Because sweat is a hypotonic solution (+/-0.3% NaCl), excess salt can build up in the body if the water lost through sweating is not replaced. Thirst cannot be relied on as a guide to the need for water; instead, water must be taken every 15 to 20 minutes in hot environments.

Under extreme conditions, such as working for 6 to 8 hours in heavy protective gear, a loss of sodium may occur. Recent studies have shown that drinking commercially available carbohydrate-electrolyte replacement liquids is effective in minimizing physiological disturbances during recovery.

Heat Collapse ("Fainting")

In heat collapse, the brain does not receive enough oxygen because blood pools in the extremities. As a result, the exposed individual may lose consciousness.

This reaction is similar to that of heat exhaustion and does not affect the body's heat balance. However, the onset of heat collapse is rapid and unpredictable. To prevent heat collapse, the worker should gradually become acclimatized to the hot environment.

Heat Rashes

Heat rashes are the most common problem in hot work environments. Prickly heat is manifested as red papules and usually appears in areas where the clothing is restrictive. As sweating increases, these papules give rise to a prickling sensation. Prickly heat occurs in skin that is persistently wetted by unevaporated sweat, and heat rash papules may become infected if they are not treated.

In most cases, heat rashes will disappear when the affected individual returns to a cool environment.

Heat Fatigue

A factor that predisposes to heat fatigue is lack of acclimatization. The use of a program of acclimatization and training for work in hot environments is advisable.

The signs and symptoms of heat fatigue include impaired performance of skilled sensorimotor, mental, or vigilance jobs. There is no treatment for heat fatigue except to remove the heat stress before a more serious heat-related condition develops.

EXPOSURE LIMITS

The risk of heat-induced illnesses depends on the individual sensitivity to heat. Age, weight, degree of physical fitness, degree of acclimatization, metabolism, use of alcohol or drugs, and a variety of medical conditions such as hypertension all affect a person's sensitivity to heat. However, even the type of clothing worn must be considered. Prior heat injury predisposes an individual to additional injury.

The American Conference of Governmental Industrial Hygienists (1992) states that workers should not be permitted to work when their deep body temperature exceeds 38 degrees C (100.4 degrees F).

CRITERIA FOR ENTRY INTO THE MEDICAL SURVEILLANCE PROGRAM

Any worker whose work operation involves high air temperatures, radiant heat sources, high humidity, direct physical contact with hot objects, or strenuous physical activities (refer to Appendix B).

SURVEILLANCE FREQUENCY

Every worker who works in extraordinary conditions that increase the risk of heat stress should be personally monitored. These conditions include wearing semipermeable or impermeable clothing when the temperature exceeds 21 degrees C (69.8 degrees F), working at extreme metabolic loads (greater than 500 kcal/hour), etc.

Personal monitoring can be done by checking the heart rate, recovery heart rate, oral temperature, or extent of body water loss.

To check the heart rate, count the radial pulse for 30 seconds at the beginning of the rest period. If the heart rate exceeds 110 beats per minute, shorten the next work period by one third and maintain the same rest period.

The recovery heart rate can be checked by comparing the pulse rate taken at 30 seconds (P (1)) with the pulse rate taken at 2.5 minutes (P (3)) after the rest break starts. The two pulse rates can be interpreted using Table 10-1.

Table 10-1: HEART RATE RECOVERY CRITERIA

HEART RATE RECOVERY CRITERIA

Heart Rate Recovery Pattern	P(3)	Differences between P(1) and P(3)
Satisfactory Recovery	< 90	---
High Recovery (Conditions require further study)	90	10
No Recovery (May indicate too much stress)	90	< 10

Oral temperature can be checked with a clinical thermometer after work but before the employee drinks water. If the oral temperature taken under the tongue exceeds 37.6 degrees C, shorten the next work cycle by one third.

Body water loss can be measured by weighing the worker on a scale at the beginning and end of each workday. The worker's weight loss should not exceed 1.5% of total body weight in a workday. If a weight loss exceeding this amount is observed, fluid intake should increase.

Fluid Replacement

Cool (50-60 degrees F) water or any cool liquid (except alcoholic beverages) should be made available to workers to encourage them to drink small amounts frequently, e.g., one cup every 20 minutes. Ample supplies of liquids should be placed close to the work area. Although some commercial replacement drinks contain salt, this is not necessary for acclimatized individuals because most people add enough salt to their summer diets.

Table 10-2: Requirements For Heat Stress For Extremely Hot Environments

Requirements For Heat Stress For Extremely Hot Environments	
Pre-placement exam	Yes
Periodic exam	Yes - Annually
Emergency/exposure Examination and Tests	No
Termination exam	No
Examination includes special emphasis on these body systems	Cardiovascular and Respiratory
Work and medical history	Yes
Chest x-ray	No
Pulmonary function test (PFT)	No
Other required tests	EKG
Evaluation of ability to wear A respirator	No
Additional Tests if deemed necessary	
Written medical opinion	Yes
Employee counseling re: exam results, Conditions of increased risk	No
Medical removal plan	Yes

Chapter 11: Lasers

The term "LASER" is an acronym for "Light Amplification by Stimulated Emission of Radiation." A laser is device that emits a highly collimated beam of intense monochromatic radiation when energized. The spectrum of electromagnetic radiation ranges from the ultraviolet region through the visible to the infrared region. Laser radiation may be emitted as a continuous wave or as pulses.

A continuous wave (cw) is the output of a laser which is operated in a continuous rather than a pulsed mode. The American National Standard (ANSI) Z136.1-1986 states a laser operating with a continuous output for a period ≥ 0.25 s is regarded as a cw laser.

Maximum permissible exposure (MPE) is the level of laser radiation to which person may be exposed without hazardous effect or adverse biological changes in the eye or skin. The criteria for MPE for the eye and skin are detailed in ANSI Z136.1-2000 Safe Use of Lasers for exposure limits.

EXPOSURE LIMITS

Maximum Permissible Exposure values established by the ANSI for Safe Use of Lasers. The level of laser radiation to which a person may be exposed without hazardous effects or adverse biological changes in the eye or skin. Refer to ANSI Z136.1-2000 Safe Use of Lasers for exposure limits.

CRITERIA FOR ENTRY INTO THE MEDICAL SURVEILLANCE PROGRAM

Medical Surveillance is only necessary for the following laser classes:

Class IIIb Laser - a moderate powered laser (cw of 5.0 - 500.0 mw; pulsed, 10 J/cm2). In general, Class IIIb lasers will not present a fire hazard and are not generally capable of producing a hazardous diffuse reflection. Specific controls including mandatory Personal Protective Equipment (PPE) are recommended.

Class IV Laser - a high-powered laser (cw of >500.0 mw) which is hazardous to view under any condition (directly or diffusely scattered) and is a potential fire and skin hazard. Significant controls are required of Class IV laser systems and facilities.

Medical surveillance shall be provided to employees using Class IIIb or IV lasers and associated equipment. The company's Medical Surveillance Request Form will be mailed from EHS to the supervisor upon request. Users shall return the completed form to EHS.

Upon receiving the medical surveillance form, EHS will schedule an appointment for the employee with an occupational health physician.

PHYSICAL EXAMINATION

A one-time ophthalmology exam is required. If the employee passes the exam, no further examinations are necessary unless deviations occur. However, following any suspected laser injury, the pertinent examinations will be repeated (refer to Appendix H).

Table 11-1: Requirements For Laser Operators

Requirements For Laser Operators	
Pre-placement exam	Yes – An one time initial vision/color depth
Periodic exam	A yearly laser information sheet
Emergency/exposure Examination and Tests	Yes
Termination exam	No
Examination includes special emphasis on these body systems	Eyes
Work and medical history	No
Chest x-ray	No
Pulmonary function test (PFT)	No
Other required tests	No
Evaluation of ability to wear A respirator	No
Additional Tests if deemed necessary	No
Written medical opinion	Yes
Employee counseling re: exam results, Conditions of increased risk	Yes
Medical removal plan	No

About the Author

Thomas M. Socha is the Senior Project Manager at People Technology, Inc., located in Rochester Hills, Michigan. Mr. Socha has a Master of Science in Hazardous Waste Management from Wayne State University, Detroit, Michigan.

Appendix

APPENDIX A–Medical Surveillance Request Form

ENVIRONMENTAL HEALTH AND SAFETY MEDICAL SURVEILLANCE REQUEST FORM	RETURN FORM TO: Office Of Environmental Health and Safety or	
NAME:	SSN:	SEX:
HOME ADDRESS:	HOURS WORK PER WEEK:	DATE OF BIRTH:
DEPARTMENT:	WORK PHONE:	
JOB TITLE:	DEPARTMENT FAX NO.:	
SUPERVISOR:	SUPERVISOR PHONE:	

CHECK TYPE OF EXAMINATION(S) REQUESTED):

	Respirator Use – Reason for respirator use:
	Heat Stress – Reason for heat stress:
	Noise Exposure – Reason for noise exposure:
	Aerial Work Platform Operator (aerial lift)
	Animal Handler – Animal Handler Code(s)
	Blood Borne Pathogens
	TB Testing every year (Health Care Workers)
	Laser Operator (Class IIIB or Class IV lasers)
	Other-Please be Specific:

Supervisor Authorization Signature:

MEDICAL EXAM DESCRIPTIONS

Exam Type	Employees Who Need Exam	Frequency of exam
Respirator Use	Wearing a respirator while performing work tasks	1-3 years (determined by a physician)
Heat Stress	Performing strenuous physical work in an environment with high air temperature, high humidity, radiant heat or direct contact with hot objects	Annual
Noise Exposure	Working in high noise environments	Annual
Aerial Work Platform Operator	Operating an aerial work platform device	Questionnaire Only
Animal Handler	Employees who handle small animals more 8 hours per week, or have incidental contact/handle large animals	See reference Codes
TB Testing – every year	Employees that work as Health Care Workers are require to be TB tested annually	Annual
Blood Borne Pathogens		None (see guidelines)
Laser Operator	Operators of Class IIIB or Class IV lasers	One time initial exam
Other – Please be specific	If you have a situation that should be evaluated	

73

APPENDIX B–General Health Questionnaire

GENERAL HEALTH HISTORY QUESTIONNAIRE

Name:		SSN:	Date of Exam:
Address:		Birthdate:	Sex: M F
		Work Tel:( )	
City:	State:	Home Tel( )	
Zip Code:		Job Title	

2. HEALTH HISTORY

Yes No	Yes No	Yes No
Any surgery or hospitalization in last 5 years?	Shortness of breath	Spinal injury or disease
Any serious illness in last 5 years requiring medical attention?	Lung disease, emphysema, asthma, chronic bronchitis, pleurisy	Chronic, severe low back pain
Head/Brain injuries, disorders or illnesses	Kidney disease, dialysis	Regular, frequent alcohol use
Seizures, epilepsy	Liver disease	Narcotic or habit forming drug use
medication	Digestive problems	
Eye disorders or impaired vision (expect corrective lenses)	Diabetes or elevated blood sugar controlled by diet medication insulin	
Ear disorders, loss of hearing or balance	Nervous or psychiatric disorders, e.g., serve depression	
Heart disease or attack; other cardiovascular condition medication	Loss of or altered consciousness Fainting, dizziness	
Heart surgery (valve replacement/bypass, angioplasty, pacemaker)	Sleep disorders, daytime sleepiness, severe snoring	
High blood pressure medication	Stroke or paralysis	
Muscular disease	Missing or Impaired hand, arm, foot, leg, finger, toe	

For any YES answer, indicate onset date, diagnosis, medication, treating physician's name and address, any current limitation

List any other medications, not already given above, used regularly or recently.

Medical Examiner's Comments on Health History

APPENDIX C–Pre-Placement/Surveillance Results Form

	Pre-Placement/Surveillance Fitness for Duty Evauation Results Form
NAME:	SSN:
EMPLOYER:	DEPARTMENT:
JOB TITLE:	DATE OF EXAM:

Results of Pre-Placement/Surveillance/Fitness for Duty Evaluation:

    Able to work in the above job with no restrictions.
    Able to work in the above job with the following restrictions:

    Unable to work in the above job.
    Recommendation deferred pending:

Results of Respirator Evaluation:

    Able to use respirator.
    Able to use a respirator with the following restrictions:

    Unable to use a respirator.
    Respirator use deferred pending:

    Recommended next Respirator Evaluation in: 1   2   3   years (circle one)

Results of Audiometric Evaluation:

    Baseline audiogram
    Employee has incurred a threshold shift.   Left ear   Right ear
Repeat audiometric evaluation within two weeks.   Date scheduled:
Employee has not incurred a threshold shift.
Recommend follow up for additional evaluation.
Not medically able to use hearing protection.

Other:

Physician signature: Date:

APPENDIX D–Zoonoses Questionnaire

CONFIDENTIAL MEDICAL INFORMATION

SIGNIFICANT BIOLOGICAL AGENT OR ANIMAL CONTACT HEALTH SURVEILLANCE QUESTIONNAIRE

Return to: Medical Director, Employee Health Services

Date:_____
Chart #:_____

Name:_____Birth date:_____
Medical Record Identifier:_____

Previous Evaluation at Student Health or Employee Health? ☐ Yes ☐ No

Department:_____Recharge Number:_____Phone:_____

Status: ☐ Faculty   ☐ Veterinarian   ☐ Research Technician
        ☐ Student   ☐ Biologist   ☐ Microbiologist
        ☐ Animal Handler   ☐ Pathologist   ☐ Other

What species of animals or types of biological agents will you be handling?

Medical History

Do you have any ongoing medical problems? If yes, explain.

Have you had (check all that apply)?:

☐ Pneumonia   ☐ Recurrent Bronchitis   ☐ Tuberculosis
☐ Heart Disease   ☐ Rheumatic Fever   ☐ Heart murmur & Valve Disease
☐ Diabetes   ☐ Kidney Disease   ☐ Liver Disease
☐ Cancer   ☐ Gastrointestinal Disorder ☐ Loss of Consciousness
☐ Seizures   ☐ Arthritis   ☐ Chronic Back or Joint Pain

Have you been told by a physician that you have an immune compromising medical condition or are you taking medications that impair your immune system (steroids, immunosuppressive drugs, or chemotherapy)?_____If yes, explain_____

Are you currently taking any medications?_____If yes, list_____

For Women: Are you pregnant, or planning to be pregnant in the next year?
☐ Yes, ☐ No

Allergy History

List any allergies to medications:

Do you have any of the following symptoms (Check all that apply)?:

☐Chronic cough ☐Asthma   ☐Itchy, irritated eyes
☐Hay fever   ☐Skin rash   ☐Chronic allergies (food, pollens, dust)

Are you allergic to?

☐Dog   ☐Cat   ☐Cattle   ☐Horse   ☐Bird (feathers)
☐Hog   ☐Primates   ☐Rabbit   ☐Goat   ☐Sheep (wool)
☐Rat or mice ☐Guinea Pig   ☐Alfalfa   ☐Weeds   ☐Trees
☐Grasses   ☐Chemicals   ☐Latex   ☐Wood   ☐Other_____

Immunizations

Indicate date of most recent vaccination (or blood test to document immunity). Mark "X" if you do not recall the date. Mark "?" or leave blank if you are unsure.
Measles_____Mumps_____Rubella_____Hepatitis A_____
Hepatitis B_____Rabies_____CMV_____Toxoplasmosis_____
"Q" Fever_____BCG_____Vaccinia ("smallpox")_____
Yellow Fever_____

Date of last tetanus booster:_____

Date of last rabies booster:_____

Date of last rabies titer:_____

Date of last serum sample:_____

Tuberculosis Skin Testing

Date of last PPD skin test:_____ ☐Positive, ☐ Negative
If POSITIVE, date of last Chest X-ray:_____
If POSITIVE in the past, are you having any of the following symptoms (check box)?

☐ Fever ☐ Chronic cough ☐ Bloody sputum ☐ Weight loss ☐ Shortness of breath

Have you ever contracted a disease from animals, or experienced an animal related injury (including bites, scratches, needlesticks, etc)? If yes, please explain below:

Do you work with species of, or biological material from, **non-human primates?**
☐Yes ☐No

Are you involved with recombinant DNA technology?☐ Yes ☐ No. If yes, does the research involve techniques in which viable, recombinant DNA-containing micro-organisms are used to infect animals that then require Biosafety level 3 containment?

APPENDIX E–Respirator Medical Evaluation Questionnaire

OSHA RESPIRATOR MEDICAL EVALUATION QUESTIONNAIRE			
To the employee: Can you read (circle one):		Yes	No
Your employer must allow you to answer his questionnaire during normal working hours, or at a time and place that is convenient to you. To maintain your confidentiality, you employer or supervisor must not look at or review your answers, and your employer must tell you how to deliver or send this questionnaire to the health care professional who will review it.			
Part A. Section 1.			
The following information must be provided by every employee who has been selected to use any type of respirator (please print)			
1. Today's date:		2. Your Name:	
3. Year Age (to nearest year)		4. Sex (circle one): Male	Female
5. Your height : Ft: In.		6. Your Weight: Lbs	
7. Your Job Title:			
8. A phone number where you can be reached by the health care professional who reviews this questionnaire (include the Area Code): ( ) -			
9. The best time to phone you at this number:			
10. Has you employer told you how to contact the health care professional who will review this questionnaire (circle one):		Yes	No
11. Check the type of respirator you will be use (you can check more than one category):			
11a. N, R, or P disposable respirator (filter-mask, non-cartridge type only).			
11b. Other type (for example, half- or full-facepiece type, powered-air purifying, supplied-air or self contained breathing apparatus.			
12. Have you worn a respirator (circle one). If "yes", what type(s):		Yes	No
Part A Section 2.			
Questions 1 through 9 below must be answered by every employee who has been selected to use any type of respirator (please circle "yes" or "no").			
1. Do you currently smoke tobacco, or have you smoked in the last month:		Yes	No
2. Have you ever had any of the following conditions?			
2a. Seizures (fits):		Yes	No
2b. Diabetes (sugar disease):		Yes	No
2c. Allergic reactions that interfere with your breathing:		Yes	No
2d. Claustrophobia (fear of closed-in places):		Yes	No
2e. Trouble smelling odors:		Yes	No
3. Have you ever had any of the following pulmonary or lung problems?			
3a. Asbestosis		Yes	No
3b. Asthma		Yes	No
3c. Chronic bronchitis		Yes	No
3d. Empysema:		Yes	No

3e. Pneumonia:	Yes	No
3f. Tuberculosis:	Yes	No
3g. Silicosis	Yes	No
3h. Pneumothorax (collasped lung)	Yes	No
3i. Lung Cancer	Yes	No
3j. Broken ribs:	Yes	No

4. Do you currently have any of the following symptoms of pulmonary or lung illness?		
4a. Shortness of breath:	Yes	No
4b. Shortness of breath when walking fast on level ground or walking up a slight hill or incline	Yes	No
4c. Shortness of breath when walking with other people at an ordinary pace on level ground:	Yes	No
4d. Have to stop for breath when walking at your own pace on level ground:	Yes	No
4e. Shortness of breath when washing or dressing yourself:	Yes	No
4f. Shortness of breath that interferes with your job:	Yes	No
4g. Coughing that produces phlegm (thick sputum):	Yes	No
4h. Coughing that wakes you early in the morning:	Yes	No
4i. Coughing that occurs mostly when you are lying down:	Yes	No
4j. Coughing up blood in the last month.	Yes	No
4k. Wheezing:	Yes	No
4l. Wheezing that interferes with your job:	Yes	No
4m. Chest pain when you breathe deeply:	Yes	No
4n. Any other symptoms that you think may be related to lung problems:	Yes	No

5.Have you ever had any of the following cardiovascular or heart problems?		
5a. Heart attack:	Yes	No
5b. Stroke:	Yes	No
5c. Angina:	Yes	No
5d. Heart failure:	Yes	No
5e. Swelling in your legs or feet (not caused by walking):	Yes	No
5f. Heart arrhythmia (heart beating irregularly):	Yes	No
5g. High blood pressure:	Yes	No
5h. Any other heart problem that you've been told about:	Yes	No

6. Have you ever had any of the following cardiovascular or heart symptoms?	Yes	No
6a. Frequent pain or tightness in your chest:	Yes	No
6b. Pain or tightness in your chest during physical activity:	Yes	No
6c. Pain or tightness in your chest that interferes with your job:	Yes	No
6d. In the past two years, hsve you noticed your heart skipping or missing a beat:	Yes	No
6e. Heartburn or indigestion that is not related to eating:	Yes	No
6f. Any other symptoms that you think may be related to heart or circulation problems:	Yes	No
7. Do you currently take medication for any of the following problems?		
7a. Breathing or lung problems:	Yes	No
7b. Heart trouble:	Yes	No
7c. Blood pressure:	Yes	No
7d. Seizures (fits):	Yes	No
8. If you've used a respirator, have you ever had any of the following problems? (If you've never (if you've never used a respirator, check the following space _____ and go to question 9:)		
8a. Eye irritation:	Yes	No
8b. Skin allergies or rashes:	Yes	No
8c. Anxiety:	Yes	No
8d. General weakness or fatigue:	Yes	No
8e. Any other problem that interferes with your use of a respirator:	Yes	No
9. Would you like to talk to the health care professional who will review this questionnaire about your answers to this questionnaire?	Yes	No
Questions 10 to 15 below must be answered by every employee who has been selected to use either a full-facepiece respirator or a self-contained breathing apparatus (SCBA). For employees who have been selected to use other types of respirators, answering these questions is voluntary		
10. Have you ever lost vision in either eye (temporarily or permanently):	Yes	No
11. Do you currently have any of the following vision problems?		
11a. Wear contact lenses:	Yes	No
11b. Wear glasses:	Yes	No
11c. Color blind:	Yes	No
12. Have you ever had an injury to your ears, including a broken ear drum:	Yes	No

13. Do you currently have any of the following hearing problems?		
13a. Difficulty hearing:	Yes	No
13b. Wear a hearing aid:	Yes	No
13c. Any other hearing or ear problem:	Yes	No
14. Have you ever had a back injury:	Yes	No
15. Do you currently have any of the following musculoskeletal problems?		
a. Weakness in any of your arms, hands, legs, or feet:	Yes	No
b. Back pain:	Yes	No
c. Difficulty fully moving your arms and legs:	Yes	No
d. Pain or stiffness when you lean forward or backward at the waist:	Yes	No
e. Difficulty fully moving your head up or down:	Yes	No
f. Difficulty fully moving your head side to side:	Yes	No
g. Difficulty bending at your knees:	Yes	No
h. Difficulty squatting to the ground:	Yes	No
i. Difficulty climbing a flight of stairs or a ladder carrying more than 25 lbs:	Yes	No
j. Any other muscle or skeletal problem that interferes with using a respirator:	Yes	No

APPENDIX F–Aerial Platform Questionnaire

	Aerial Platform Questionnaire
Name:	SSN:
Address:	Home Phone:
	Date of Birth:
Employer Name:	Shift:
	Department:
Job Title:	Work Phone:

MEDICAL HISTORY

		Yes	No
1.	Have you ever been in the hospital as a patient? If yes, what kind of problems were you having?	Yes	No
2.	Have you ever had any kind of operation? If yes, what kind?	Yes	No
3.	Do you take any kind of medicine regularly? If yes, what kind?	Yes	No
4.	Have you ever been under the care of a physician during the past year? If so, for what condition?	Yes	No
5.	Have you ever been told that you had high blood pressure/	Yes	No
6.	Have you ever had a heart attack or heart trouble?	Yes	No
7.	Have you ever been diagnosed with diabetes?	Yes	No
8.	Have you ever had a seizure or convulsion?	Yes	No
9.	Do you have acrophobia (fear of heights)?	Yes	No
10.	Please explain any "Yes" answers:		
11.	Do you have any other health conditions or concerns not covered by these questions? If yes, please explain:	Yes	No

Patient Signature   Date:

APPENDIX G–Formaldehyde Questionnaire

	Formaldehyde Questionnaire (Appendix D, 1910.1028)
Name:	SSN:
Address:	Home Phone:
	Date of Birth:
Employer Name:	Shift:
	Department:
Job Title:	Work Phone:

MEDICAL HISTORY

1.	Have you ever been in the hospital as a patient? If yes, what kind of problems were you having?	Yes	No
2.	Have you ever had any kind of operation? If yes, what kind?	Yes	No
3.	Do you take any kind of medicine regularly? If yes, what kind?	Yes	No
4.	Are you allergic to any drugs, foods, or chemicals? If yes, what kind of allergy is it?	Yes	No
5.	What causes the allergy? Have you ever been told that you have asthma, hayfever, or sinusitis?	Yes	No
6.	Have you ever been told that you have emphysema, bronchitis, or any other respiratory problems?	Yes	No
7.	Have you ever been told you had hepatitis?	Yes	No
8.	Have you ever been told that you had cirrhosis?	Yes	No
9.	Have you ever been told that you had cancer?	Yes	No
10.	Have you ever had arthritis or joint pain?	Yes	No
11.	Have you ever been told that you had high blood pressure?	Yes	No
12.	Have you ever had a heart attack or heart trouble?	Yes	No

Medical History Update

1.	Have you been in the hospital as a patient any time within the past year?	Yes	No
2.	Have you been under the care of a physician during the past year? If so, for what condition?	Yes	No
3.	Is there any change in your breathing since last year? Better? Worse? No Change? If change, do you know why?	Yes Yes Yes Yes	No No No No
4.	Is your general health different this year from last year? If different, in what way?	Yes	No
5.	Have you in the past year or are you now taking any medication on a regular basis? Name Rx: Condition being treated	Yes	No

Occupational History

1.	How long have you worked for your present employer?		
2.	What jobs have you held with this employer? Include job title and length of time in each job		
3.	In each of these jobs, how many hours a day were you exposed to chemicals?		
4.	What chemicals have you worked with most of the time?		
5.	Have you ever noticed any type of skin rash you feel was related to your work?	Yes	No
6.	Have you ever noticed any type of skin rash you feel was related to your work? Wheeze? Become short of breath or cause your chest to become tight?	Yes Yes Yes	No No No
7.	Are you exposed to any dust or chemicals at home? If yes, what kind?	Yes	No
8.	Have you ever been under the care of a physician during the past year? If so, for what condition?	Yes	No
9.	Have you ever been told that you had high blood pressure/	Yes	No
10.	Have you ever had a heart attack or heart trouble?	Yes	No

Occupational History Update

1. How long have you worked for your present employer?

2. What jobs have you held with this employer? Include job title and length of time in each job

3. In each of these jobs, how many hours a day were you exposed to chemicals?

4. What chemicals have you worked with most of the time?

5. Have you ever noticed any type of skin rash you feel was related to your work?   Yes   No

6. Have you ever noticed any type of skin rash you feel was related to your work?   Yes   No
    Wheeze?   Yes   No
    Become short of breath or cause your chest to become tight?   Yes   No

7. Are you exposed to any dust or chemicals at home?   Yes   No
    If yes, what kind?

8. In other jobs, have you ever had exposure to: Yes   No
    a) Wood dust?   Yes   No
    b) Nickel of chromium?   Yes   No
    c) Silica (foundry, sand blasting)?   Yes   No
    d) Arsenic or asbestos?   Yes   No
    e) Organic solvents?   Yes   No
    f) Urethane foams?   Yes   No

Miscellaneous

1. Do you smoke?   Yes   No

    Pipe   Cigars   Cigarettes
    If so, how much and for how long?

2. Do you drink alcohol in any form?   Yes   No

    If so, how much, how long, and how often?

3. Do you wear glasses or contact lenses?   Yes   No

4. Do you get any physical exercise other than that required to do your job?   Yes   No

    If so, explain:

5. Do you have any hobbies or "side jobs" that require you to use chemicals, such as   Yes   No
    furniture stripping, sand blasting, insulation ormanufacture of urethane foam, furniture,
    etc?
    If so, please describe, giving type of business or hobby, chemicals used and length of
    exposures.

Symptoms Questionnaire

1.	Do you ever have any shortness of breath?	Yes	No
	If yes, do you have to rest after climbing several flights of stairs?	Yes	No
	If yes, if you walk on the level with people your own age, do you walk slower than they do?	Yes	No
	If yes, if you walk slower than a normal pace, do you have to limit the distance that you walk? If yes, do you have to stop and rest while bathing or dressing?	Yes	No
		Yes	No
2.	Do you cough as much as three months out of the year?	Yes	No
	If yes, have you had this cough for more than two years?	Yes	No
	If yes, do you ever cough anything up from chest?	Yes	No
3.	Do you ever have a feeling of smothering, unable to take a deep breath, or tightness in your chest?	Yes	No
	If yes, do you notice that this on any particular day of the week?	Yes	No
	If yes, what day or the week?	Yes	No
	If yes, do you notice that this occurs at any particular place?	Yes	No
	If yes, do you notice that this is worse after you have returned to work after being off for several days?	Yes	No
4.	Have you ever noticed any wheezing in your chest?	Yes	No
	If yes, is this only with colds or other infections?	Yes	No
	Is this caused by exposure to any kind of dust or other material?	Yes	No
	If yes, what kind?		
5.	Have you noticed any burning, tearing, or redness of your eyes when you are at work? If so, explain circumstances:	Yes	No
6.	Have you noticed any sore or burning throat or itchy or burning nose when you are at work? If so, explain circumstances	Yes	No
7.	Have you noticed any stuffiness or dryness of your nose?	Yes	No
8.	Do you ever have swelling of the eyelids or face?	Yes	No
9.	Have you ever been jaundiced?	Yes	No
	If yes, was this accompanied by any pain?	Yes	No
10.	Have you ever had a tendency to bruise easily or bleed excessively?	Yes	No
11	Do you have frequent headaches that are not relieved by aspirin or tylenol?	Yes	No
	If yes, do they occur at any particular time of the day or week?	Yes	No
	12.2 If yes, when do they occur:		

12.	Do you have frequent episodes of nervousness or irritability?	Yes	No
13.	Do you tend to have trouble concentrating or remembering?	Yes	No
14.	Do you ever feel dizzy, light-headed, excessively drowsy or like you have been drugged?	Yes	No
15.	Does your vision ever become blurred?	Yes	No
16.	Do you have numbness or tingling of the hands or feet or other parts of your body?	Yes	No
17.	Have you ever had chronic weakness or fatigue?	Yes	No
18.	Have you ever had any swelling of your feet or ankles to the point where you could not wear your shoes?	Yes	No
19.	Are you bothered by heartburn or indigestion?	Yes	No
20.	Do you ever have itching, dryness, or peeling and scaling of the hands?	Yes	No
21.	Do you ever have a burning sensation in the hands, or reddening of the skin?	Yes	No
22.	Do you ever have cracking or bleeding of the skin on your hands?	Yes	No
23.	Are you under a physician's care?	Yes	No
	If yes, for what are you being treated?		
24.	Do you have any physical complaints today?	Yes	No
	If yes, explain?		
25.	Do you have other health conditions not covered by these questions?	Yes	No
	If yes, explain:		

APPENDIX H–Laser Medical Surveillance Results Release Record

LASER MEDICAL SURVEILLANCE RESULTS RELEASE RECORD

RETURN COPY TO: Office of Environmental Health and Safety

Laser Permit Holder:	Department:
EXAMINEE:	SSN

DESCRIPTION OF LASER(S) (or see attached information.)

Location	Type	Class	Power	Wavelength(s)

PURPOSE OF EXAMINATION

PRE-ASSINGMENT   TERMINATION OR TRANSFER FROM LASER CONTROL AREA

TYPE OF EXAMINATION

LASER PERSONNEL   INCIDENTAL PERSONNEL

MEDICAL FITNESS STATUS OF EXAMINEE (*Completed by Physician or Physician's Representative*) The applicant has successfully completes a medical eye examination. As indicated by the type of examination above, the examination did not reveal any abnormalities that precludes laser work as a personnel or access to laser control areas as an incidental personnel.

Restrictions/Comments:

NAME:	SIGNATURE:	DATE:

ADDRESS:

I hereby authorize   Eye Center to release my to Office Environmental Health and Safety, all medical information including test results and measurements from the Laser Safety Eye Examination rendered to me on (month/date/year):

Patient Signature:	Date:
Witness Signature:	Date:

Notes

1. Title 29, Code of Federal Regulations, Part 1910.1001, *Asbestos*, current edition.

2. Title 29, Code of Federal Regulations, *Hazardous Waste Operations and Emergency Response*, Current edition.

3. Department of Labor. *OSHA Technical Manual Directive (TED 1.15) Section V*, Chapter 3, Controlling Occupational Exposure to Hazardous Drugs.

4. Center of Disease Control. *Guidelines for preventing the transmission of tuberculosis in health care facilities, 1994*. MMWR 1994; 43 (No. RR-13): 1-132.

5. Hunt LW, Fransway AF, Reed CEE, et al. *An epidemic of occupational allergy to latex involving health care workers*. Journal Occupational Environmental Medince 1995; 37:1204-1209.

6. CDC, Update provisional public health service recommendations for chemoprophylaxis after occupational exposure to HIV. MMWR 1996; 45(22) 468-480.

7. CDC. *Mumps prevent*. MMWR 1989; 38: 288-92, 397-400.

8. Lemon SM, Thomas DL. *Vaccines to prevent viral hepatitis*. New England Journal of Medicine 1997: 336: 196-204.

9. CDC. Prevention and control of influenza. *Recommendations of the immunization practices advisory committee (ACIP)*. MMWR 1996; 45(RR-5): 1-24.

10. Sullivan JB, Kriger GR, editors. *Hazardous materials toxicology*. Baltimore: Williams and Wilkins. 1992.

11. *Control of Communicable Diseases in Man*. Beneson AS(ed). Washington DC: American Public Health Association, 1995, p. 165-7.

12. California Environmental Protection Agency. Office of Environmental Health Hazard Assessment. *Guidelines for physicians who supervise workers exposed to cholinesterase-inhibiting pesticides.* 3rd edition 1995.

13. Hayes WJ. *Pesticides studied in man.* Baltimore: Williams and Wilkins, 1982. P.309.

14. Section 651 et seq. of Title 29, United States Code, *Occupational Safety and Health Act of 1970,* as amended.

15. Lawry RR, Hoet P. *Industrial Chemical Exposure*: Guidelines for biological monitoring. 2nd ed Boca Raton: Lewis Publishers, 1993: 25 6-59.

BIBLIOGRAPHY

American Conference of Governmental Industrial Hygienists (ACGIH). *1992-1993 Threshold Limit Values for Chemical Substances and Physical Agents and Biological Exposure Indices.* Cincinnati: American Conference of Governmental Industrial Hygienists.

Arizona State University, *Laser Medical Surveillance Results Release Record.*

Department of Defense Occupational Health Surveillance Manual, May 1998. *https://www.denix.osd.mil/denix/Public/ES-Programs/Safety/Documents/6055.5/manual.html.*

Department of Labor, OSHA. Title 29, Code of Federal Regulations, Part 1910.95, *Occupational Noise Exposure*, Current Edition

Department of Labor, OSHA. Title 29, Code of Federal Regulations, Part 1910.134, *Respiratory Protection*, Current Edition.

Department of Labor, OSHA. Title 29, Code of Federal Regulations, Part 1910.1030, *Bloodborne Pathogens*, Current Edition

Department of Labor, OSHA. Title 29, Code of Federal Regulations, Part 1910.1048, *Formaldehyde*, Current Edition.

Department of Labor, Occupational Safety and Health Administration (OSHA). *Screening and Surveillance: A Guide to OSHA Standards, OSHA 3162.* 1999.

Department of Labor. *OSHA Technical Manual Directive (TED 1.A15) Section II*, Chapter 2, Heat Stress.

Oakland University, *Respiratory Safety Program*, Current Edition

Oakland University, *Bloodborne Pathogens Exposure*, Current Edition

University of California at Davis. *Occupational Health Issues in Care and Use of Research Animals.* *http://clueless.ucdavis.edu/health/OccHealthBackground.html*

University of Michigan, Occupational Safety and Environmental Health (OSEH). *Medical Surveillance Program* website. *http://www.umich.edu/~oseh/occmed.html.*

University of Michigan, University Committee on Use and Care of Animals. *Unit for Laboratory Animal Medicine.* *http://www.research.umich.edu/ULAM/PAGES/UCUCA/HLTHPAMF.HTM*

University of Missouri–Columbia, *The Business Policy and Procedure Manual*, Chapter: Health and Safety, Section 7:020, "Health and Medical Surveillance Program–Animal Care Personnel," May 27, 1994. *http://www.pmn.missouri.edu/mubussrv/07-020.html.*

INDEX

Made in the USA
Lexington, KY
02 March 2015